Psychiatric and Mental Health Nursing Certification

Nancy Randolph, RN, MSN, CS, CNAA

Springhouse Corporation
Springhouse, Pennsylvania

Staff

Executive Director, Editorial
Stanley Loeb

Publisher, Trade and Textbooks
Minnie B. Rose, RN, BSN, MEd

Art Director
John Hubbard

Senior Editor
David Moreau

Drug Information Editor
George J. Blake, RPh, MS

Associate Acquisitions Editor
Betsy Snyder

Copy Editors
Diane M. Armento, Pamela Wingrod

Designers
Stephanie Peters (associate art director), Donald G. Knauss, Mary Stangl

Manufacturing
Deborah Meiris (manager), T.A. Landis, Anna Brindisi

Printed in the United States of America.

PSY-010293

Library of Congress Cataloging-in-Publication Data

Randolph, Nancy
American nursing review for psychiatric and mental health nursing certification / Nancy Randolph.
p. cm.
Includes bibliographical references and index.
1. Psychiatric nursing — Outlines, syllabi, etc.
2. Psychiatric nursing — Examinations, questions, etc. I.Title
[DNLM: 1. Psychiatric Nursing — examination questions. WY 18 R194a 1993]
RC440.R33 1993
610.73′68′076 — dc20
DNLM/DLC   92-48438
ISBN 0-87434-513-8   CIP

Contents

Contributors

EXECUTIVE CLINICAL EDITOR

Nancy Randolph, RN, MSN, CS, CNAA
Director, Center of Nursing
Jersey Shore Medical Center
Neptune, New Jersey

CONTRIBUTORS

Ann Clarke Berkery, RN, MS, CS
Nurse Psychotherapist and Clinical Nurse Specialist
Private practice
Berkeley Heights, New Jersey

Carol J. Bininger, RN, PhD
Assistant Professor
College of Nursing
Ohio State University
Columbus, Ohio

Mary K. Collins, RN, MSN, CS
Associate Professor
University of Rochester
Rochester, New York

Dierdre D. Fisher, RN, MSN, CS, CNA
Director, Education and Practice
New Jersey State Nurses Association
Trenton, New Jersey

Margery G. Garbin, RN, PhD
President
C-NET
Martinsville, New Jersey

Kathleen M. Gialanella, RN, JD
Attorney-at-law
Gutterman, Wolkstein, Klinger & Yohalem
Westfield, New Jersey

Deborah R. Oestreicher, RN, MS, CS
Nurse Psychotherapist
Private practice
Piscataway, New Jersey

Margaret H. Pipchick, RN, MA, CS
Clinical Specialist, Psychiatric Nursing
Private practice
Cranford, New Jersey

Nancy Randolph, RN, MSN, CS, CNAA
Director, Center of Nursing
Jersey Shore Medical Center
Neptune, New Jersey

Foreword

As a discipline matures and the theoretical base for practice expands, specialization is inevitable and necessary. Even the most complicated situations become understandable and manageable when seen through the eyes of practitioners who have focused their knowledge and experience on one specialty. At the same time, expansion of knowledge and subsequent maturation of the field can only occur at the point of specialization. Scientific inquiry must proceed inductively, carefully studying specialized situations and eventually allowing new insights to filter down to generalist practice. In a manner of speaking, specialization is both the means and the end of an evolving discipline.

This process has allowed learned disciplines and professions to protect specialty practice from governmental control or external regulation. Instead, they have chosen to impose strict standards from within. Appreciating the sophisticated knowledge necessary for problem solving in these specialized situations, society has deferred to the professions' internal mechanisms.

Certification — the bridge between internal and external control — serves three important functions. First, it holds members of the profession accountable for a standard of practice. Second, it serves the profession by allowing the cognitive richness of the discipline to grow unencumbered. Third, it serves the public by providing visible proof of an individual's qualifications to practice in a designated specialty area.

More than 220,000 nurses are currently certified through 30 organizations. The rapid growth of this voluntary personal credential is testimony to organized nursing's intent to honor its stewardship to the public while ensuring the growth of the field.

Programs of certification have moved along a circuitous route to their current status and prominence. Reviewing the chain of events from the early 1950s to 1974, when the first national certification examination was given, creates a healthy respect for organizational politics and for the principle that form follows function. The concept of certification in the health care fields was originally pioneered by medicine and introduced to nursing as early as 1945 by the American Association of Nurse Anesthetists (AANA). Certification took on a seriousness in the late 1950s, as the American Nurses Association (ANA) established the goal of developing mechanisms for "formal recognition of personal achievement and superior performance in nursing." Although the intent of creating a personal credential to recognize competence in specialty practice was clearly expressed, progress was hampered by an ANA organizational structure driven by functional roles rather than clinical specialization.

From the late 1950s to the mid 1970s, informal conference groups were established around clinical specialty areas until the divisions on clinical practice became a permanent part of the ANA structure. In planning for this change, the ANA initially recognized 13 clinical practice designations but subsequently recognized only five broadly defined divisions. Although economics was purportedly the reason for these structural choices, the association's leaders had philosophical disagreements about the ANA's primary mission. The controversy focused on whether the ANA should have an authoritative role in monitoring the standard of services that nurses render to the public and whether it should claim to speak for specialized groups in clinical practice. Eventually, divisions were charged with developing standards, disseminating information to their peers, and certifying in their areas of practice. A new organizational form evolved, one that valued the contribution of specialized clinical practice. This became necessary to accommodate a field in which scientific growth depended on the clinical practice environment.

The first national certification examination was administered in 1974, 16 years after the ANA originally committed to create a credential for specialized practice. Internal competition for limited resources and continuing philosophical conflicts over program priorities seriously hampered further progress. These same conflicts mitigated against the creation of structural units that would appeal to the increasingly finite specialty interests of nurses. The broad clinical areas recognized by the ANA proved inadequate to the needs of evolving practice. In response, specialty societies formed outside the ANA.

Even if ANA organizational politics moved slowly, the public demand for quality assurances in health care did not, and the government sometimes responded by addressing specialty practice issues when adequate internal regulation by the professions did not exist. In New Jersey in February 1971, a governmental certification for marriage counselors jeopardized the right of nurse-psychotherapists to practice. Although this situation was challenged politically, it sensitized nursing to the need to recognize the practice competency of its own members. With unprecedented speed, the clinical specialists of the New Jersey State Nurses Association (NJSNA) developed a certification process, obtained a board of nursing interpretation that this credential would signify an individual's competence to practice as a nurse-psychotherapist, and established the Society of Certified Clinical Specialists under the Psychiatric Mental Health Nursing Practice Division of the NJSNA. The first certified nurses were recognized in May 1972. This accomplishment of New Jersey nurses is testimony to a singularity of purpose, an openness to compromise and negotiation, and the power of a critical mass of nurses motivated to monitor their practice on behalf of the public.

Exposed to similar governmental pressure, the New York State Nurses Association (NYSNA) established a comparable certification program in 1973, signaling a relationship between NYSNA and NJSNA that would grow closer in the ensuing years. The significant overlapping membership of these state associations and the mobility across state borders resulted in mutual recognition of the New York and New Jersey certifications and collaboration on examination development. The certification process consisted of a credentials review, paper-and-pencil examination, and evaluation of case material. Over time, the case material requirement was deleted, and the ANA certification examination was accepted as the paper-and-pencil component. However, experiential requirements focusing on the nurse-psychotherapist role still sets this credential apart.

The integration of this certification program within NJSNA has yielded various insights and benefits. The decision to recognize ANA's certification for clinical specialists in adult psychiatric mental health nursing resulted in an appreciation that the New Jersey certification signified competence as a nurse-psychotherapist rather than as a clinical specialist. Members of the Society became trailblazers for the state nursing association's accomplishments in reimbursement and clinical privileges, and they established a legal defense fund and a continuing education institute. As the Society and the nurse-psychotherapist certification in New Jersey celebrate their 20th year, they remain firmly integrated in the professional association, committed to guaranteeing the integrity of their service, and consistently available to stand with one another against all challenges.

Lucille A. Joel, RN, EdD, FAAN
President, American Nurses Association
Charter Member, Society of Certified Clinical Specialists in Psychiatric Nursing, NJSNA

Preface

Certification in psychiatric and mental health nursing is professional recognition of a nurses's high achievement of specialty knowledge and superior nursing practice. It is a signal to both professional peers and the public of a nurses's advanced qualifications in psychiatric and mental health nursing practice.

In her foreword to this book, Lucille Joel, president of the American Nurses Association (ANA) from 1988 to 1992, provides a historical perspective of the certification movement in nursing from the 1940s to the present day. Thousands of nurses now take the certification examination each year. As the public continues to demand more quality assurance, high standards of health care, and professional accountability, the number of certified nurses will continue to increase.

Nurses who take the ANA's certification examination must demonstrate superior knowledge of psychiatric and mental health nursing and the ability to apply that knowledge to a wide variety of psychiatric clients in varied health care settings. To pass the test, the nurse must resharpen test-taking skills and develop new strategies for answering a different style of test question from what the nurse may remember appearing on the "State Boards" many years ago.

This first-ever review book on psychiatric and mental health nursing certification has been designed to help nurses pass the ANA's Psychiatric and Mental Health Nursing Certification Examination. It contains all the elements needed to:
- understand how the examination is developed and scored
- develop successful test-taking skills and strategies
- complete a thorough review of psychiatric nursing concepts, theories, and practices
- evaluate readiness to take the actual examination.

Chapter 1 describes the eligibility requirements for taking the test and reviews the examination blueprint. Knowing what is likely to be on the examination is fundamental to knowing what to study. To give the nurse a framework for building self-confidence, the chapter also offers proven test-taking strategies, analyzes the structure of test questions, and provides hints for selecting the correct answer.

Chapter 2 reviews concepts central to understanding basic human emotional responses, from anxiety to anger to grief. Chapter 3 explores human development. Chapter 4 reviews the ever-expanding settings, roles, and scope of psychiatric and mental health nursing practice. Chapter 5 focuses on theoretical models of human behavior. Chapter 6 reviews the techniques of gathering, manipulating, and reporting research data, an important component of advanced practice.

Chapter 7 covers therapeutic communication, one of the primary tools of psychiatric and mental health nursing practice. Chapter 8 explains the essential legal aspects of nursing practice, such as informed consent, confinement, and clients' rights.

Chapters 9 to 17 cover the major psychiatric disorders seen by psychiatric and mental health nurses. The text reviews etiology, signs and symptoms, possible nursing diagnoses, and nursing interventions. Additionally, the text presents relevant diagnostic criteria from the *Diagnostic and Statistical Manual of Mental Disorders*, Third Edition, Revised (perhaps better known by its abbreviated name, *DSM-III-R*). Each of these chapters also includes a clinical situation (case study) based on one of the disorders discussed in that chapter. Organized around the nursing process, the clinical situation examines the client's health problems through the phases of assessment, diagnosis, planning, implementation, and evaluation. Rationales for each nursing action (in italic type) give the reader a complete foundation for planning nursing care.

Chapter 18 reviews the individual, group, and rehabilitative therapies commonly used to treat psychiatric disorders, including their purpose, indications for use, and nursing implications.

Chapter 19 covers the major drug groups used in psychiatric treatment: antipsychotic agents, antiparkinsonian agents, tricyclic antidepressants, monoamine oxidase (MAO) inhibitors, antimanic agents, benzodiazepines, and sedative-hypnotic agents. For each group, the text presents indications, mechanism of action, pharmacokinetics, adverse effects, contraindications, and nursing implications. Tables for each group provide information about specific pharmaceutical products.

The post-test, written in the same format used on the actual examination, covers all study areas that appear in the certification blueprint. Correct answers and rationales follow, along with a diagnostic profile, to give the nurse a reliable indication of which areas require further study.

Three appendices provide information for additional preparation: the ANA's standards of psychiatric and mental health nursing practice, the 1992 NANDA-approved taxonomy of nursing diagnoses, and normal values for common laboratory tests. Selected references offer opportunities for further study and research, and the index serves as a handy guide when trying to locate a topic quickly.

American Nursing Review for Psychiatric and Mental Health Nursing Certification contains all the information a nurse needs to prepare successfully for the psychiatric and mental health nursing certification exam. I hope that this book helps you in your quest for certification and that you use it as a reference in your practice for many years.

F. William Balkie, RN, MBA, CRNA
President
American Nursing Review

1 Certification examination

In 1973, the American Nurses Association (ANA) established a certification program in psychiatric and mental health nursing to recognize the expert knowledge and practice of psychiatric nurses. The largest of all ANA certification programs, it has certified more than 12,000 nurses to date.

The ANA offers three examinations for psychiatric nursing certification: a basic psychiatric and mental health nurse examination, a clinical specialist examination for adult psychiatric and mental health nursing, and a clinical specialist examination for child and adolescent psychiatric and mental health nursing. Administered by the American Nurses Credentialing Center (ANCC) each June and October in cities throughout the United States and its territories, the examinations are given in the morning and last about 3 hours.

Eligibility and application

The ANCC establishes criteria for eligibility to take the examination. Requirements for the basic examination differ from those of the clinical specialist examinations. The criteria discussed in this book were in effect as of the 1992 examination. Because requirements can change, candidates should obtain the latest criteria before applying for certification (see *Certification eligibility requirements*, pages 2 and 3).

Once you have decided to prepare for the examination, you may want to obtain the certification catalog by writing the American Nurses Credentialing Center, 600 Maryland Avenue S.W., 100 West, Washington, DC 20024, or by calling toll free, 1-800-284-2378. This catalog provides all the information you will need to apply.

Be sure to pay careful attention to all steps in the application process. Failure to complete any step correctly may make you ineligible to take the examination on the date you had planned. All applicants must pay a nonrefundable application fee and an examination fee, set each year by the credentialing center.

Certification test plan

After establishing your eligibility, the credentialing center will mail you a handbook that contains the current examination blueprint, or test plan. This test plan delineates the test content and the ratio (weighting) of each content area for that particular test. Information about the test plan, especially its content, can provide considerable guidance in helping you organize your study plan.

In recent years, the basic examination in psychiatric and mental health nursing has included such topics as *assessment* (physical examination, health and development history, psychosocial assessment, mental status examination), *problem identification and planning* (health care team meetings, coordination of interdisciplinary treatment measures, identification of nursing diagnoses, establishment of treatment goals), *intervention* (therapeutic milieu, treatment

Certification eligibility requirements

The American Nurses Credentialing Center's eligibility criteria for certification in psychiatric and mental health nursing, in effect as of 1992, are listed below. Note that the requirements for the basic examination differ from those of the specialist examinations.

Criteria for a psychiatric and mental health nurse
By the time of application, you must:
A. Hold an active RN license in the United States or its territories
B. Have practiced as a licensed registered nurse in direct psychiatric and mental health nursing practice for 24 of the past 48 months and must have engaged in direct psychiatric and mental health nursing for a minimum of 1,600 hours
C. Be involved in direct psychiatric and mental health nursing practice for an average of 8 hours/week
D. Have access to clinical consultation or supervision
E. Submit a reference from a nurse colleague on Form B, obtained from the ANA (If the nurse is not from your place of employment, you must submit an additional reference from a non-nurse mental health colleague from your place of employment on Form C. This reference is based on any arrangement that allows psychiatric and mental health nurses to discuss their work in an ongoing way with an experienced mental health colleague.)
F. Have had 30 contact hours of continuing education applicable to the specialty area in the past 3 years (Presenter, lecturer, and participant credits are allowable. However, presenter or lecturer credits can account for no more than one-half of the credits. A combination of continuing education and academic credit hours is acceptable. Contact-hour credit is allowed for attendance at professional meetings that include content appropriate to psychiatric and mental health nursing practice. Independent study that has been approved for continuing education or academic credit also is allowed.)

Criteria for a clinical specialist in adult or child and adolescent psychiatric and mental health nursing
By the time of application, you must:
A. Hold an active RN license in the United States or its territories
B. Be currently involved in direct psychiatric and mental health nursing practice for an average of 4 hours/week
C. Have access to clinical consultation or clinical supervision
D. Have experience in at least two different treatment modalities
E. Have educational preparation that meets one of three criteria:
　1. Hold a master's or higher degree in nursing with specialization in psychiatric and mental health nursing
　2. Hold a master's or higher degree in nursing outside the psychiatric and mental health nursing field with a minimum of 24 graduate or postgraduate academic credits in psychiatric and mental health theory and supervised clinical training in two psychotherapeutic treatment modalities
　3. Hold a master's or higher degree in a mental health field that included a minimum of 24 graduate or postgraduate academic credits in psychiatric and mental health theory and supervised clinical training in two psychotherapeutic treatment modalities (This option ends after the 1993 test administration. Individuals who receive their first license as reg-

Certification eligibility requirements *(continued)*

istered nurses in 1990 and thereafter must hold a baccalaureate in nursing if their
master's or higher degree is in a nonnursing mental health field.)

F. Have 2 years of post-master's-degree practice in psychiatric and mental health nursing with a
minimum of 8 hours/week of direct client contact, or 4 years of post-master's-degree practice in psychiatric and mental health nursing with a minimum of 4 hours/week of direct client contact

G. Document 100 post-master's-degree hours of individual, group, or peer group clinical consultation and receive an endorsement from the consultant or supervisor

    1. The consultation may include, but is not limited to, any group of two or more nurses eligi-
ble for certification as clinical specialists in psychiatric and mental health nursing who
meet regularly (such as 1 hour/week, 4 hours/month, 12 hours/quarter) and consult
via case reviews, telephone, mail, audiotapes, videotapes, and so forth. Creative alternatives are encouraged in order to help nurse colleagues meet this requirement.

    2. The endorsement must be provided by a qualified consultant or supervisor

        a. Clinical specialist in psychiatric and mental health nursing

            (1) ANCC-certified clinical specialist in psychiatric and mental health nursing

            (2) Clinical specialist with a master's degree in psychiatric and mental health nursing

            (3) Clinical specialist with a master's or higher degree in nursing outside the psychiat-
ric and mental health nursing field who meets the certification requirements

        b. Individual with advanced preparation in psychiatry or psychology (qualifies as a con-
sultant or supervisor only through the 1993 test administration)

            (1) A master's-prepared psychiatric social worker

            (2) A psychiatrist

            (3) A psychologist prepared at the doctoral level and listed in the National Register of
Health Service Providers in Psychology

            (4) A psychologist prepared at the doctoral level in an APA-accredited program in
clinical psychology, counseling psychology, or school psychology

---

approaches, comprehensive teaching, crisis intervention), *evaluation* of nursing
care, and *professional issues* (client advocacy, nursing research).

The clinical specialist examinations have included such topics as *treatment*
(psychotherapeutic interventions, health training, self-care, somatic treatment,
therapeutic environment, psychotherapy), *education* (education of others, continuing self-education), *research* (participation, communication), *management*,
and *consultation*.

According to the certification catalog, all parts of the nursing process and interdisciplinary collaboration will be represented in examination items within the
appropriate content category.

The certification examination is developed by the Board on Certification for
Psychiatric and Mental Health Nursing Practice. The test objectively evaluates
knowledge, comprehension, and application of psychiatric nursing theory and
practice to client care. The committee defines the content areas covered in each
test and the emphasis placed on each area.

Certified psychiatric and mental health nurses from around the country contribute questions for each examination. The test-development committee reviews each test item for accuracy, readability, and relevance to the test plan. Sample questions approved by the committee are compiled into an examination that will be used on the next test date.

Each test contains approximately 150 multiple-choice questions, usually preceded by brief clinical situations. Candidates have 3 hours to complete the test. A break is usually provided, but this may vary from year to year.

Test results are mailed to all candidates about 3 months after the examination. No results are released early or over the telephone to protect the privacy of candidates.

Preparing for the certification examination

To ensure success on the examination, you must know how to analyze questions and use specific strategies to help you select the best response. Readiness for taking the test involves three areas of preparation: intellectual, physical, and emotional.

Intellectual preparation includes a complete review of all the subjects that will be covered on the test. This book provides you with an organized source for that review. Supplement its use with other sources, such as current medical and nursing literature, particularly if the subject is not one you deal with every day in your practice. If you take a review course, pay special attention to unfamiliar material being discussed, and be sure to ask the instructor for clarification when necessary. You also may want to discuss topics covered in the review course with other participants or perhaps organize a study group to review difficult material after the course is over.

Finally, take the post-test included in this book; then review the correct answers and analyze your performance by completing the accompanying diagnostic profile. The post-test will expose you to questions from all content areas covered on the certification examination, and the diagnostic profile will help you pinpoint the reasons for incorrect answers, thereby suggesting areas for further study to help you avoid repeating these mistakes on the actual test.

Physical preparation for the examination may seem obvious, but many candidates ignore its importance. Staying up all night before the test to cram last-minute information is an obvious mistake. Sound physical preparation also involves applying to take the test well in advance and securing all the necessary documents to ensure your eligibility. Keep your test permit in a safe place, and remember to take it with you to the examination. If you live near the examination site, visit it in advance to gauge travel time and familiarize yourself with parking facilities. Nothing can affect your performance more adversely than arriving late in a state of high anxiety. Make overnight reservations early if you have to travel a long distance. Staying close to the test location will promote a good night's sleep and prompt arrival. If you are sensitive to room temperature, plan to take a sweater; it's easy to put on or remove quickly. Take mints or hard candy to relieve a dry mouth. Finally, eat a light but nourishing breakfast. It will give you the energy you need to perform at an optimum level.

Emotional preparation markedly influences test performance. Be confident. Think positively. Look at the examination as a way of demonstrating your mastery of the subject matter. After all, you have been practicing psychiatric nursing for many years. You have a wealth of knowledge about most of the test content. You have taken standardized tests before, the most memorable being the NCLEX-RN (State Boards). Everyone feels anxious before an important examination. The feeling is normal, even beneficial. All psychiatric nurses know that mild anxiety keeps you alert, motivates you to study, and helps you to concentrate. However, you also know that too little or too much anxiety can affect performance. Think about past experiences when you have been anxious during a test. If you recall being too anxious, now is the time to learn some simple relaxation exercises, such as rhythmic breathing or progressive muscle relaxation. Guided imagery, such as imagining yourself successfully answering all the questions on the test, can be helpful. Remind yourself of those relaxation techniques that worked in the past. They can work again. During the test, avoid becoming distracted by others who may be exhibiting anxious behavior. Concentrate on the test in front of you, and keep your feelings under control. Positive feelings will help you relax and keep your confidence high. Don't be bothered by people who seem to have finished the test early. Tell yourself that they have just given up and probably did not complete the exam.

Test-taking strategies

You can improve your chances of passing standardized multiple-choice examinations by using techniques that have proven successful for others. These techniques include knowing how timed examinations are administered, understanding all the parts of a test question, and taking specific steps to ensure that you have selected the correct answer.

Time management becomes crucial when taking a standardized test, because the candidate receives no credit for unanswered questions. Consequently, you should try to pace yourself to finish the test on time. Remember, you'll have about 1 minute to answer each question. Don't spend too much time on any one question. Instead, place a light pencil mark next to it and come back later, if time is available. Other questions may stimulate your recall of the correct answer for the question you left unanswered. Also, keep in mind that you will not be penalized for guessing. If you have no idea of the correct answer, select any option; you still have a 25% chance of being correct.

All questions on the certification examination have been carefully crafted and pretested to ensure readability and uniformity. Understanding the components of a question can help you analyze what it is asking, which will increase the likelihood that you will respond correctly. The diagram on the next page shows the parts of a multiple-choice question. Note how clearly the question is written, with no unnecessary words in the stem. Each option is relatively uniform in length. (See *Parts of a test question,* page 6.)

Read every question carefully. If a clinical situation precedes the question, study the information given. Watch for key words (such as *most, first, best,* and *except*). They are important guides to which option you should select. For example, if a question reads, "Which of the following nursing actions should the nurse perform first?", you may find that all of the listed options are appropriate for the client's condition, but only one of them clearly takes precedence over the others.

Parts of a test question

Multiple-choice test questions on the certification examination are constructed according to strict psychometric standards. As shown below, each question has a stem, four options, a key (correct answer), and three distractors (incorrect answers). A brief clinical situation, or case study, usually precedes the questions.

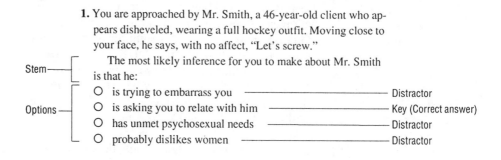

As you read the stem, try to anticipate the correct answer. Look at the options to see if your answer is listed. If so, it's probably the correct one.

If you do not see your expected answer in the options, read all the options again before you select one. If you select an option before reading all of them, you'll deny yourself the opportunity to evaluate all the choices. Try to find an option that most closely resembles the one you thought would be correct. If you don't find one, look for the best option available. Remember, you're looking for the best answer among those given. It may not be what you think is the best response, but it's all you have to work with.

For some questions, you may see two options that seem correct and you can't decide between them. Look at them again. There has to be a difference. Read the stem again. You may discover something that you didn't see before that will help you make a selection. If not, and you still can't choose, make an educated guess, and place a light mark by the question so you can return to it later.

Despite thorough preparation, you may not know the answer to some questions. Relax. Remember that you are an expert practitioner; you possess a wealth of information. Think of client cases that you have had, and recall information about them that you can apply to the question. Tell yourself the principle involved, and recall what you know about applying that principle to practice situations. At the very least, this will help you eliminate some of the options that are probably wrong. Now you have narrowed the selection process down to perhaps two options. This should make your choice easier.

If time still remains when you answer the final item, return to questions that you marked for later review or did not answer. Erase the mark and answer the question, or review your answer for possible change. Do not be afraid to change a selection if you think of a better choice later. Finally, remember to erase any marks in your test book that do not belong there. Your examination will be scored by computer, and extraneous marks could affect the scoring.

Taking the certification examination shows confidence in your knowledge about psychiatric nursing. Following an organized study program, such as the one provided in the following pages, will help ensure that you are fully prepared to take the test.

2 Fundamental concepts

I. Anxiety

A. Anxiety is a universal, subjective feeling of vague, generalized apprehension

B. This emotion is crucial to human survival, yet excessively high levels of anxiety can interfere with one's ability to maintain health

C. Four theories of anxiety hold special importance for psychiatric and mental health nursing

    1. In the late 19th century, with his *psychodynamic theory,* Sigmund Freud first discussed a psychological basis for anxiety

        a. Anxiety signals the ego of an emerging unconscious impulse

        b. Anxiety is a key emotion of the ego, indicating hidden psychological conflicts

    2. According to the *learned theory,* which was first proposed about 1977 by A. Bandura and others, anxiety is a learned response to an unpleasant stimulus

        a. Avoiding the unpleasant stimulus reduces anxiety

        b. The person ultimately learns to avoid unpleasant stimuli

    3. The *biochemical theory,* which evolved from the work of many theorists from 1977 to 1980, proposes that high anxiety levels correlate with increases in heart rate, blood lactase level, and oxygen use during moderate exercise

        a. These changes increase midbrain activity, which releases norepinephrine

        b. Increased norepinephrine in humans increases anxiety

    4. In 1986, Isaac Marks formulated the *genetic theory*

        a. All organisms, including humans, are selectively bred for defensive behavior

        b. Autonomic susceptibility to threats is genetically determined

D. Anxiety falls under one of four categories

    1. *State anxiety* is transient apprehension that fluctuates in intensity and that is usually related to a specific situation or occurrence

    2. *Trait anxiety* is a permanent characteristic marked by strong, frequent bouts of anxiety from precipitating stressors, such as threats to self-esteem or physical safety

> **3.** *Acute anxiety* is an intense physical and psychological episode that occurs without warning and that causes a sense of impending doom
>
> **4.** *Chronic anxiety* is a fixed part of one's personality that is manifested by nervousness, insomnia, and continual irritability

E. An individual can experience four levels of anxiety

   1. *Mild anxiety* is a normal state of tension characterized by alertness; enhanced concentration and perception; a sharpened ability to think, reason, and learn; and a high level of motivation resulting in organized and focused behavior

   2. *Moderate anxiety* narrows one's focus, causing the individual to ignore or block out selective parts of what caused the anxiety level to rise; characteristics include selective attention, reduced perception and concentration, diminished thinking and problem-solving abilities, and behavior that focuses on the immediate interest

   3. *Severe anxiety* markedly reduces one's ability to cope with life's events because the individual focuses totally on a specific event to the exclusion of everything else; characteristics include markedly narrowed perception, loss of concentration, internally directed attention to relieve distress from the anxiety, and severely reduced thinking, reasoning, and problem-solving abilities

   4. *Panic anxiety* is an extreme maladaptive response to stress characterized by greatly impaired perception; complete disorganization of the personality; inability to reason, solve problems, or think rationally; and complete inability to function safely without help

F. Anxiety is manifested psychologically, physically, and cognitively

   1. *Psychological symptoms* include a feeling of impending doom, decreased perception, loss of control, tension, nervousness, and withdrawal from others

   2. *Physical symptoms* include syncope; shortness of breath; heart palpitations; a "lump" in the throat; sweating, especially in the palms; and nausea or "butterflies"

   3. *Cognitive symptoms* include loss of attention, reduced ability to solve problems, impaired concentration, inability to make decisions, and reduced work productivity

II. Stress

A. Stress is any biopsychosocial external or internal experience that one views as demanding, challenging, and threatening

B. Stress is a dynamic process that contributes to personal survival and growth or behavioral dysfunction and death

C. In 1950, Hans Selye advanced the study of stress theory by articulating the Generalized Adaptation Syndrome (GAS)

   1. Selye identified three stages of stress response in humans

      a. The *alarm reaction* mobilizes the body's defense resources against a real or perceived threat

      b. The body begins to adapt through increased *resistance* to the stressor

      c. *Exhaustion* occurs when the body's resources are depleted and cannot resist the stressor

   2. These responses, based on Selye's postulates, may be adaptive or maladaptive

   3. One's ability to recognize stress is crucial to the success of stress management

D. Stressors usually occur in groups over time; the number of stressors and the time they occur influence one's ability to cope with them

   1. In 1967, Holmes and Rahe developed a list of "stressful life events"; ranked according to the coping behavior required of a person, the top 10 stressors are death of a spouse, divorce, marital separation, jail term, death of a close family member, personal injury or illness, marriage, termination from employment, marital reconciliation, and retirement

   2. More recent studies by Cassel, Cobb, and Caplan suggest that the magnitude of life changes resulting from the stressor is more important than the stressor itself

   3. Other research shows that the dissatisfactions with and problems of everyday life accumulate over time and ultimately have a greater effect on mental well-being than specific stressors

E. Human response to stress depends on one's perception of the stressor, available coping resources, intellectual and emotional states, and sense of well-being

   1. How a person responds to stress can be affected by physiologic, psychological, and sociocultural factors

      a. Physiologic factors include one's genetic makeup, nutritional status, and overall health

      b. Psychological factors include innate intelligence, self-esteem, sense of self-control, and morale

      c. Sociocultural factors include one's age, educational preparation, occupation, and economic status

   2. The psychophysiologic signs of stress are the same as those of anxiety (see Section I-F on page 9)

F. Health education and individual client teaching can mitigate the effects of stress; commonly used stress management techniques include meditation, biofeedback, relaxation exercises, and stress-inoculation training

III. Anger

A. One of the primary human emotions, anger is a feeling of displeasure that occurs when one perceives a threat; the resulting tension must be released to avoid physical or psychological harm

1. When expressed externally, anger is marked by aggression that can vary from mild indignation to violent rage
2. Anger can be released in positive or negative ways
   a. Positive releases of anger include developing increased motivation to achieve, making changes, and developing confidence in other opinions
   b. Negative releases of anger include cursing, using sarcasm, closing out further communication, and physical assault
3. Anger can be expressed internally or externally
   a. Internal expression of anger may produce increased heart rate and respiratory rate, hyperactivity, tension, or hostility
   b. External expression of anger may produce assertiveness, passivity, aggression, acting-out behavior, or rage

B. Theories of anger have their roots in the fields of biology, psychology, and sociology
   1. Biological theories of anger include the instinctual drive theory and the neurobiological theory
      a. According to the *instinctual drive theory,* anger is an innate drive common to all animals
      b. According to the *neurobiological theory,* neurotransmitters deep in the brain activate anger from other neural stimulation
   2. Psychological theories of anger include the frustration-aggression theory and the behavioral theory
      a. According to the *frustration-aggression theory,* a blocked or unattainable desire results in frustration, which causes aggressive behavior
      b. According to the *behavioral theory,* aggression is learned early in life because it helps achieve goals
   3. Sociocultural theories of anger include the social learning theory and the social environment theory
      a. According to the *social learning theory,* social behavior developed through interacting with others teaches aggression
      b. According to the *social environment theory,* expressions of anger are based on the social environment in which one lives; lack of personal territory increases aggressive behavior

C. An individual can successfully manage anger by responding directly to the problem, by using assertiveness training techniques, and by setting reasonable limits on behavior
   1. Direct response refers to an individual's conscious effort to reduce tension by engaging in physical activity (for example, taking a brisk walk alone or playing tennis or racquetball)
   2. Assertiveness training — a planned, conscious process to deal positively with anger — involves concrete steps
      a. Analyze personal behavior
      b. Record situations of assertive behavior

      c. Observe how others react in similar situations

      d. Identify alternative ways to handle situations

      e. Try new alternatives

      f. Get feedback on performance from others

    3. Setting limits helps prevent unreasonable expressions of anger that intrude on others

      a. State acceptable boundaries of behavior

      b. Assist the person to express reasons for the anger

      c. Develop alternative behaviors

IV. Grief

A. Grief is a powerful emotional reaction to a separation or loss, such as declining health, impending death, the death of a loved one, or the loss of a valuable personal object

B. Expressions of grief vary considerably, depending on one's personality, cultural background, and intensity of feeling toward the loss

C. Healthy grieving is time limited, becoming less intense as time passes but taking 1 year or more to resolve fully

D. Grief can have physical, psychological, and social ramifications

    1. Physical signs include insomnia; tight muscles, especially in the throat and chest; interrupted sleep; loss of appetite; and lethargy and generalized weakness

    2. Psychological signs include preoccupation with or ambivalence toward the lost object; anger; fantasies that the object is not lost; and guilt over inability to prevent the loss

    3. Social signs include withdrawal from usual social activities and decreased work productivity

E. Healthy grieving consists of three stages: realization, disorganization, and resolution

    1. In stage I (realization), shock, disbelief, and numbness initially overwhelm the person

      a. The individual becomes angry and resentful when others offer support

      b. The individual uses inner resources in an attempt to regain the lost object

      c. The stage ends when the person gradually accepts the irreversibility of the loss

    2. In stage II (disorganization), emotional pain from realization of the permanence of the loss creates disorganized behavior, loneliness, and a profound sense of helplessness

      a. The person develops guilt over what could have been done to prevent the loss

      b. Crying, preoccupation with the lost object, despair, and loss of interest in social interactions are magnified

3. In stage III (resolution), the bereaved person begins to think about life without the lost object

    a. Emotional pain decreases, as evidenced by less crying and preoccupation with the loss

    b. The person starts to develop a new life-style, focusing on new objects and new purposes for living

F. Dysfunctional grieving results from ambivalence toward the lost object, intolerance of the emotional pain of grieving, and social isolation; it requires professional interventions

    1. Help the client experience the emotions of grieving by exploring the importance of the lost object

    2. Encourage the client to recall memories of the lost object in order to identify and express the loss

    3. Encourage the client to express all feelings about the loss, even negative ones

    4. Encourage the client to develop independent relationships with others to talk about the loss in his or her own terms

    5. Teach the client how the grieving process functions

    6. Help the client develop goals for the future by focusing on individual strengths and abilities

V. Coping

A. Coping is an individualized effort to understand and handle life's problems

B. Everyone develops resources to cope with stressors

    1. The amount of coping effort required depends on how one evaluates the threat of the stressor in relation to one's inner coping abilities

    2. Understanding a client's appraisal of life's stressors and the coping resources developed is crucial to providing individualized nursing care

    3. The coping resources that people use (first described by Mechanic, Lazarus, and Folkman) include individual skills and abilities, social support, economic resources, motivation, defensive techniques, personal health, and high self-esteem

C. Coping mechanisms are the person's efforts to reduce stress and anxiety

    1. An individual may cope with mild anxiety through outbursts of temper, crying, vigorous exercise, fantasizing, or sleeping

    2. More severe levels of anxiety, which become ego threatening, require more extreme coping efforts, such as the use of ego-centered defense mechanisms

        a. *Compensation* — emphasizing a perceived asset to make up for a perceived liability

        b. *Denial* — ignoring and refusing to recognize the reality of what is occurring in a person's life

    c. *Displacement* — transferring a feeling from an actual object or person to a more neutral one

    d. *Dissociation* — breaking off part of the personality from the rest of one's consciousness

    e. *Identification* — adopting the attributes of another person who is admired or perceived as an authority figure

    f. *Intellectualization* — using excessive cognition to ignore an unpleasant feeling

    g. *Projection* — attributing one's unacceptable thoughts or desires to another

    h. *Rationalization* — using excuses to justify undesirable behavior or thinking

    i. *Reaction formation* — demonstrating behavior that directly opposes one's true feelings

    j. *Regression* — reverting personality development to an earlier functional level

    k. *Repression* — removing undesirable thoughts or impulses from conscious awareness

    l. *Sublimation* — substituting an undesirable trait or impulse for one that is more socially acceptable

    m. *Substitution* — using an alternative source of satisfaction for one that is not available

3. Destructive behavioral patterns dispel anxiety without resolving the cause

    a. *Neurotic behavior* — evidenced by distressing symptoms without socially unacceptable behavior and no reality testing impairment

    b. *Psychotic behavior* — characterized by a disintegrated personality, regressive behavior, disturbances in affect, and gross impairment of reality testing

VI. Transference and countertransference

A. *Transference* refers to a client's idealization of the therapist during psychotherapy

    1. Client feelings toward the therapist originate from feelings the client had toward a significant other earlier in life

    2. Transference is revealed during therapy and can help the client in clarifying reality

    3. Two types of transference can intrude on a nurse-client relationship

        a. In *hostile transference,* the client directs hostility and rage internally by becoming discouraged with the therapeutic progress or externally by criticizing the therapist's capabilities

        b. In *dependent-reaction transference,* the client becomes submissive and adoring and views the therapist as all-knowing and wise

    B. *Countertransference* refers to projection of the therapist's feelings about a significant other to the client during therapy

        1. Many clients provoke emotional reactions in the therapist

        2. The therapist may respond to these feelings through emotion or behavior that is inappropriate for and incongruent with the reality of the therapeutic situation

            a. Love reactions — involving one's self in the personal or social life of the client

            b. Hostile reactions — showing anger or arguing with the client

            c. Anxiety reactions — feeling guilty, uneasy, or nervous when interacting with the client

        3. Countertransference can be therapeutically harmful and must be quickly addressed by the therapist

VII. Crisis and crisis intervention

    A. *Crisis* refers to an imbalance in internal equilibrium that results from a stressor or threat to the self

        1. Crises develop from perceived or real losses, such as the death of a loved one, a job loss, or new challenges

        2. A crisis usually consists of four phases

            a. In phase I, a precipitating event occurs

            b. In phase II, the ego perceives the degree of threat and tries to use previously successful coping methods

            c. In phase III, anxiety builds, thinking becomes disorganized, and the person develops a sense of helplessness

            d. In phase IV, the person organizes personal resources, tries new coping methods, or redefines the threat in a way that renders previously learned problem-solving techniques effective

        3. An individual may experience one of three types of crisis

            a. Maturational crises are normally occurring events in life caused by the person's continual growth and development

            b. Situational crises are unexpected events (such as job loss or a loved one's death) that disrupt the biopsychosocial balance

            c. Social or adventitious crises are major cataclysmic disasters (such as an earthquake, flood, or war) that cause a massive upheaval of social and personal order

    B. *Crisis intervention* aims to restore the person to a precrisis level of functioning and order; its methods resemble the phases of the nursing process

        1. Assessment consists of the following actions:

            a. Identify the precipitating event

            b. Assess the client's perception of the event

            c. Assess available coping skills and resources

         2. Analysis and planning involve the following actions:

            a. Organize assessment data

      b. Analyze the data

      c. Explore options to resolve the problem

      d. Decide on the steps needed to achieve the solution

   3. Implementation consists of the following actions:

      a. Change the client's physical situation; provide emotional support and shelter

      b. Compare the nurse's perception of the problem with the client's to clarify any misconceptions

      c. Secure economic and social resources by referring the client to appropriate help groups

      d. Acknowledge the multiple feelings a client has about the crisis to help the client sort out and express fears and expectations

      e. Help the client develop and test possible solutions

   4. Evaluation involves the following actions:

      a. Determine the effectiveness of implementations by observing behavioral outcomes and comparing them with goals

      b. Refer the client for additional help if outcomes differ from those planned

C. Crisis intervention focuses on resolving the immediate crisis and requires the nurse's active involvement in numerous techniques

   1. *Abreaction* — asking open-ended questions that will encourage the client to express emotions about the crisis

   2. *Clarification* — helping the client see the relationship between problems and the client's feelings by encouraging the client to express the cause (problem) and effect (client's reaction)

   3. *Suggestion* — guiding a client to accept a suggestion or idea that promotes self-confidence and optimism

   4. *Manipulation* — influencing a client to benefit from the therapeutic intervention by using the client's values

   5. *Reinforcement* — giving positive feedback when the client makes healthy responses to the problem

   6. *Promoting self-esteem* — communicating confidently that the client has the inner strength to find a solution to the problem

   7. *Support defenses* — assisting the client to use positive defense mechanisms that promote self-esteem and ego strength rather than maladaptive defense mechanisms that deny or impair reality

   8. *Exploring solutions* — intently examining potential solutions to the problem with the client

3 Human development

I. Overview

A. Human development proceeds in a cephalocaudal direction, from the simple to the complex

B. The developmental process is unique for each person, and what develops in the future depends on what has already happened

C. General theories of developmental behavior provide a foundation for examining the characteristics of the life cycle

D. Understanding the relative norms for important stages of development in the life cycle enables a nurse to assess whether a client has made satisfactory progress within expected boundaries

E. Theoretical models focus on the psychoanalytic, psychosocial, and cognitive aspects of human development and provide concepts that guide the delivery of nursing care

II. Psychoanalytic models of development

A. Sigmund Freud, considered the father of psychoanalysis, described psychosexual development through adolescence; his model embraces four major tenets

   1. All behavior holds some meaning about an individual's personality

   2. An individual's personality consists of three parts

      a. The *id,* the unconscious mind, operates instinctively and without control

      b. The *ego,* the conscious mind, maintains contact with reality, examining all environmental and physiologic changes experienced by the individual

      c. The *superego* is the human conscience that directs and controls thoughts and feelings

   3. To mature, an individual must successfully traverse five stages of psychosexual development

      a. During the *oral stage* (birth to 18 months), the child learns to handle anxiety by using the tongue and mouth

      b. During the *anal stage* (18 months to age 3), the child learns to control muscles, especially those controlling urination and defecation

      c. During the *phallic (Oedipal) stage* (ages 3 to 6), the child becomes cognizant of his or her sex and genitalia

d. During the *latency stage* (ages 6 to 12), the child experiences a relatively quiet phase when sexual development and energy are quiescent

e. During the *genital stage* (age 12 to adulthood), sexual interest emerges as the individual strives to develop satisfactory relations with potential sex partners

4. Unresolved conflicts at any stage of psychosexual development become fixated and remain part of the individual's personality

B. In 1963, Erik Erikson expanded on Freud's work to encompass the life cycle

1. According to Erikson's model, psychosocial development is a series of conflicts having favorable or unfavorable resolutions

2. This development occurs in eight stages (with some degree of overlap)

   a. *Trust vs. mistrust* (birth to age 1½): the child develops a sense of trust in or mistrust of others

   (1) Consistent, affectionate care during this time produces a favorable resolution

   (2) Deficient, inconsistent care produces an unfavorable one

   b. *Autonomy vs. shame and doubt* (ages 1½ to 3): the child learns self-control or becomes self-conscious and full of doubt

   (1) Praise, support, and encouragement in using newly acquired skills of independence will favorably resolve this stage

   (2) Shaming or insulting the child will cause unnecessary dependence

   c. *Initiative vs. guilt* (ages 3 to 6): the child initiates spontaneous activities or develops fear of wrongdoing

   (1) Encouraging creative activities and giving clear explanations for events occurring in the child's life promote resolution of this stage

   (2) Threatening punishment or labeling behavior as "bad" develops childhood guilt and fears of wrongdoing

   d. *Industry vs. inferiority* (ages 6 to 12): the child either develops the social and physical skills necessary to negotiate and compete in life or has feelings of inadequacy and inferiority

   (1) Recognizing the child's sensitivity and fostering activities that can be successfully completed builds confidence and resolves this stage

   (2) Unjust criticism or unreasonably high expectations will create a sense of inadequacy and inferiority

   e. *Identity vs. role diffusion* (ages 12 to 20): the teenager either integrates childhood experiences into a personal identity or develops self-doubts about sexual or occupational roles

   (1) Helping the adolescent make decisions, encouraging active participation in home events, and assisting with future plans aid resolution

        (2) Not answering questions important to the teenager and imposing unilateral control over daily activities create personality confusion

   f. *Intimacy vs. isolation* (ages 18 to 25): the person develops commitments to work and to other people or avoids close personal relationships and long-term life-style commitments

        (1) Teaching the young adult to achieve goals and foster personal relationships resolves this stage

        (2) Ridiculing romances or derogating job selection causes the young adult to withdraw and avoid friendships and career

   g. *Generativity vs. stagnation* (ages 21 to 45): the person either establishes a family and becomes creative and productive or lacks outside interests and becomes self-indulgent

        (1) Recognizing the person's responsibilities, providing emotional support, and praising achievements help resolve this stage

        (2) Failure at work, divorce, or lack of attachment to the community fosters self-indulgence and detachment from society

   h. *Integrity vs. despair* (age 45 to death): the person reviews life for meaning, fulfillment, and contributions made to the next generation or becomes dissatisfied with life, denies personal existence, and fears death

        (1) Exploring the positive aspects of one's life, such as contributions made and knowledge gained, successfully resolves this stage

        (2) Deciding that life has no meaning or purpose creates despair and hopelessness

  3. Unsuccessful passage through one stage influences passage through subsequent stages, creating the potential for psychosocial conflicts

III. Cognitive and moral models of development

  A. In 1963, Jean Piaget postulated that human development evolves from cognition, learning, knowing, and comprehending

    1. Personal maturation, socialization, and life's experiences set the course for development

    2. Cognitive development is a continuous and orderly process, occurring in four stages

      a. *Sensorimotor* (birth to 1½ years): the child learns about the self and the immediate environment by exploring, discovering objects, and imitating others

      b. *Preoperational* (ages 2 to 7): the child develops expressive language, imaginative play skills, intuitive reasoning, and the ability to explain concepts and understand dimensions of space

      c. *Concrete operations* (ages 8 to 12): the child can systematically organize thoughts and facts about the environment and begins to engage in abstract thinking

    d. *Formal operations* (age 12 to adulthood): the person can conceptualize and deal with abstractions; can hypothesize, test, and evaluate solutions to problems; develops an adult identity

B. Louis Kohlberg emphasized the development of a personal morality, proposing six stages, or orientations, of moral development

    1. *Obedience and punishment orientation:* the person obeys an authority figure and views misbehavior in terms of damage done

    2. *Instrumental relativist orientation:* the person defines "right" as that which is acceptable to and approved by the self

    3. *Intrapersonal concordance orientation:* the person maintains cordial human relations and the approval of others

    4. *Authority and duty orientation:* the person develops respect for authority and a duty to maintain the social order

    5. *Social contract orientation:* the person understands the morality of having democratically established laws

    6. *Universal ethics orientation:* the person understands the principles of human rights and personal conscience

IV. Interpersonal models of development

A. Harry Stack Sullivan theorized that interpersonal relations influenced how one's life would develop

    1. Interpersonal growth is based on satisfying basic biologic needs

    2. To form satisfactory relationships with others, one must complete six stages of development

        a. *Infancy stage* (birth to age 1½): the infant learns to rely on caregivers to meet desires and needs

        b. *Childhood stage* (ages 1½ to 6): the child learns to accept not having desires and needs met immediately

        c. *Juvenile stage* (ages 6 to 9): the child forms fulfilling relationships with peers

        d. *Preadolescence stage* (ages 9 to 12): the child successfully relates to same-sex companions

        e. *Early adolescence stage* (ages 12 to 14): the adolescent learns to be independent and to form congenial relationships with members of the opposite sex

        f. *Late adolescence stage* (ages 14 to 21): the person establishes a close, long-lasting relationship with someone of the opposite sex

B. In 1985, Daniel Stern postulated that children pass through four increasingly complex stages of self-relatedness during the first 2 years of life

    1. *Emergent self stage* (birth to 2 months): the infant begins to learn by making discriminating choices within the environment; developing awareness becomes the precursor for subsequent stages

2. *Core self stage* (2 to 9 months): the infant begins to change the focus of interpersonal relationships away from the self and toward others, usually the caregivers

3. *Subjective self stage* (9 to 18 months): the child commands attention in order to share experiences and develops the capacity to evaluate others' feelings toward self

4. *Verbal self stage* (18 to 24 months): the child develops language skills that enhance interpersonal relationships

V. Life cycle characteristics

A. Norms for growth and development usually are categorized according to widely accepted (albeit arbitrary) age ranges

B. Behavior patterns commonly overlap age ranges because each person's developmental process is unique

C. The eight age ranges, with prominent characteristics typically achieved at each range, are as follows:

1. Infant (birth to age 1½)

    a. Rapidly developing motor skills highlight the early period, with physical development proceeding cephalocaudally, proximally to distally, and from general to specific movements

    b. Social-play skills emerge, giving the infant a strong sense of self and a distinct personality with whom to relate

    c. By the end of the period, the child can express affection and sympathy and likes to initiate household chores

2. Early child, or toddler (ages 1½ to 3)

    a. The child walks and explores the ever-growing world, becomes more coordinated, dances, rides a tricycle, and has a 900-word vocabulary

    b. Socially, the child begins this period by playing alone and using temper tantrums to control others; the child also imitates older children and fears strangers and desertion by caregivers

    c. By the end of the period, the child knows and identifies with his or her own gender, plays with others, can tolerate brief separation from caregivers, and has participated in toilet training

3. Middle child, or preschooler (ages 3 to 6)

    a. Physical growth slows; fine motor skills develop, characterized by the ability to skip, throw overhand, use scissors, and tie shoelaces

    b. Socially, the preschooler plays cooperatively, bathes and dresses independently, can be rude to others, and likes to fight

    c. A developing sense of conscience begins to control initiative; the child fears wrongdoing or parental disapproval

4. Late child, or school-age child (ages 6 to 12)

    a. Physically, the child develops better motor skill control and more poise, but still is awkward in trying new activities; height and weight increase; secondary sex characteristics begin to appear later in this period

    b. The child prefers associating with same-sex companions early in this period; competes but hates to lose; and can understand what society deems as unacceptable behavior but cannot always choose between right and wrong without assistance

    c. Developing initiative and high self-esteem during this period helps the child acquire the skills needed to succeed in school

5. Adolescent (ages 12 to 20)

    a. Physically, the teenager tires easily because the cardiovascular and respiratory systems develop more slowly than the other body systems; sex characteristics blossom; dramatic physical growth produces clumsiness from failure to adapt quickly enough to physical changes

    b. Adolescents enjoy partying and building independent relationships apart from the family

    c. Uncertainty about and inexperience in the working world make career selection difficult

6. Young adult (ages 20 to 40)

    a. At the peak of physical maturity when entering this period, the young adult has minimal health concerns; energy and body function begin to diminish as the person gets older; proper nutrition, exercise, and rest help sustain well-being

    b. Marriage, family, and career create adjustments, compromise, and change while enabling the adult to realize adolescent dreams

    c. The adult sorts out values and beliefs, discarding some of those learned earlier in favor of new ones; failure to achieve personal integration causes isolation later

7. Middle adult (ages 40 to 70)

    a. Strength, physiologic reserve, and body systems continue to decline; dietary changes (for instance, less fat and more vitamins) become important; chronic diseases and sexual problems diminish self-esteem

    b. Social responsibilities widen to include parents, work associates, and neighbors; grown children leave home, creating an empty-nest syndrome

    c. Mid-life crises occur, possibly spawning divorce, substance abuse, a new occupation, or changes in the way one perceives his or her future role in life; the idealized self is replaced with a more realistic one; the person finds social value in life's accomplishments

8. Late adult (age 70 and older)

    a. Physical functioning diminishes further; muscle tone and bone density decrease; vision and hearing losses result in reduced personal mobility; diminished sense of taste causes a loss of appetite, leading to nutritional imbalance; reductions in neurologic and sensory function impair reaction time

b. Retirement from employment changes the person's role identity, social activity, finances, and living habits; the deaths of friends and family reduce social contacts unless new ones are made

c. The older adult evaluates the purpose of life and the contributions made to society; religion becomes more important as the older adult contemplates death more frequently; developing effective coping skills and a positive evaluation of one's contribution to society help create a strong sense of personal significance

4 Settings, roles, and scope of practice

I. Overview

A. Modern psychiatric nursing practice emerged in 1946 with the creation of the National Institutes of Mental Health (NIMH) and the authorization of psychiatric nursing education grants by the federal government

B. Graduate programs in psychiatric and mental health nursing proliferated throughout American universities

C. As the educational level of psychiatric nurses increased, roles expanded for practitioners and opportunities for nurses to practice in different and more varied settings increased

D. Contemporary psychiatric and mental health nursing practice in its current varied roles became official when the NIMH recognized psychiatric nursing as a legitimate mental health discipline

II. Practice settings

A. Psychiatric and mental health nurses work in a wide range of practice settings

B. Hospitals provide a client-restrictive setting where the client receives intense treatment and constant monitoring

C. Transitional facilities offer partial hospitalization and intense therapy for a client who is psychiatrically stable enough to forgo traditional hospitalization

D. Outpatient clinics provide various assessment and treatment services and typically involve just a brief stay (daily or a few hours)

E. Community mental health centers provide 24-hour emergency services, aftercare consultation and education, and treatment and rehabilitation for addiction disorders

F. The client's home serves as the practice setting for community health nurses, who visit periodically to evaluate the client's adaptation to community life and to conduct client teaching

III. Functional roles and role components

A. Psychiatric and mental health nurses provide direct care (carrying out nursing tasks) and indirect care (supervising others)

B. In 1976, the ANA Division on Psychiatric and Mental Health Nursing issued a statement on psychiatric nursing activities (see page 26)

C. Psychiatric and mental health nurses assume various roles when providing care
  1. Staff nurse
  2. Head nurse
  3. Supervisor
  4. Nursing administrator
  5. Consultant
  6. Staff educator
  7. Client advocate
  8. Clinical specialist

D. Psychiatric and mental health nurses provide a variety of major services known as role components, seven of which are universal to all practice settings
  1. Planning and implementing care through a therapeutic relationship
  2. Managing the socioenvironment
  3. Administering and monitoring drugs
  4. Assisting clients with activities of daily living
  5. Educating clients and families
  6. Facilitating family and group interaction
  7. Working with an interdisciplinary team

IV. Scope of practice

A. Psychiatric and mental health nursing practice involves working with a multidisciplinary mental health team
  1. A nurse can be a member of three classes of teams
     a. *Unidisciplinary* team members are from the same discipline
     b. *Multidisciplinary* team members are from different disciplines, each providing specific client services
     c. *Interdisciplinary* team members are from different disciplines, formally organized to provide coordinated care based on the unique contribution of each team member
  2. Nurses are commonly designated the team leader because they are always present in the client environment
  3. Mental health teams include the following:
     a. Psychiatrist, who specializes in the treatment of mental illnesses
     b. Psychiatric nurse, who specializes in managing the client environment and giving 24-hour care
     c. Clinical psychologist, who specializes in diagnostic testing of mental processes
     d. Psychiatric social worker, who specializes in family and social evaluation of the causes of client illnesses

Psychiatric nursing activities

Psychiatric and mental health nurses engage in various activities to promote the client's well-being. Primary activities recognized by the American Nurses Association include:
- providing a therapeutic milieu
- working with here-and-now problems of clients
- using the surrogate-parent role
- caring for the somatic aspects of the client's health problems
- teaching factors related to emotional health
- acting as a social agent
- providing leadership to other personnel
- conducting psychotherapy
- engaging in social and community action related to mental health.

Source: American Nurses Association, Division on Psychiatric and Mental Health Nursing Practice: *Statement on psychiatric and mental health nursing practice.* Kansas City, 1976.

    e. Psychiatric technician, who assists nurses in giving care and meeting the client's basic needs

    f. Dietitian, who specializes in developing and providing a nourishing diet for the client

    g. Occupational therapist, who specializes in assessing the client's ability to perform useful tasks that contribute to client resocialization

    h. Recreational therapist, who specializes in assessing the client's ability to engage in leisure activities (such as hobbies and sports) that contribute to the client's resocialization

    i. Spiritual advisor, who specializes in meeting the client's spiritual needs

    j. Client, who is the focus of the care plan and who participates in decisions about care if able

4. Barriers to effective team functioning can occur if individual team members' roles and functions are not agreed upon by the whole team; Benfar has described three obstacles to effective team functioning

    a. Poor identification of roles and functions

    b. Inability to resolve role overlaps

    c. Intrateam communication problems

5. For a team to work therapeutically, each member must know the following:

    a. The goals that have been established

    b. The specific therapeutic activities that will be provided

    c. The effects of therapeutic activities on the client's goals

6. The principles of collaborative (interdisciplinary) practice are:

    a. All team members focus on and contribute to the client outcomes

     b. The client participates in team meetings if able

     c. Specific functions of each discipline are unique and yet overlap with other disciplines

B. A major role of the psychiatric and mental health nurse is to provide leadership for a group

    1. The group may be a unit nursing staff, a mental health team, a quality assurance committee, or a community group

    2. An effective leader can influence group activities to achieve goals by:

     a. Communicating group goals clearly

     b. Motivating group participants to excel

     c. Initiating new ideas about how to reach group goals

     d. Helping group members express feelings and concerns

     e. Integrating the group's achievements into a greater organizational structure

    3. Primary leadership roles involve the following:

     a. *Communication* — transmitting information between two or more people and between organizational levels

     b. *Delegation* — giving responsibility to others for completing assignments

     c. *Education* — teaching others new skills and knowledge

     d. *Innovation* — being a change agent by taking risks to try new techniques and procedures to achieve goals

     e. *Control* — monitoring outcomes to ensure that goals are being met

    4. A leader typically displays one of three styles of leadership

     a. *Authoritarian style* — a rigidly structured, rule-oriented approach with the focus on the leader, who clearly is in charge

     b. *Democratic style* — collaborative direction with group members; shared decision making and member-centered focus

     c. *Laissez-faire style* — little or no direction; leaves group members to their own resources; unsure of goals

    5. Effective leadership is more likely under the following conditions:

     a. Group goals are clearly defined

     b. Group members agree on goals

     c. Goals are measurable

     d. Group goals coincide with personal and organizational goals

     e. Group expectations are clearly known

     f. Expectations are organizationally compatible

     g. Group expectations can be met

C. Quality assurance — monitoring and evaluating the quality and legitimacy of client care compared to accepted standards — also falls within the scope of nursing practice

1. Quality assurance programs ensure that high-quality care is consistently delivered to every client
   a. The programs document that standards are being met
   b. They introduce changes in care delivery based on accepted standards for objectively measuring the quality of client care
      (1) Medicare and Medicaid standards
      (2) American Nurses Association (ANA) Standards of Nursing Practice
      (3) Joint Commission on Accreditation of Healthcare Organizations (JCAHO) standards
      (4) Departments of health in each state
      (5) Individual health facility standards
   c. The focus of a quality assurance program is always on the client and the treatment plan
2. Current social and political commitments to evaluating health care are motivated by numerous groups
   a. Consumers demanding quality care
   b. Third-party payers (insurance companies) desiring cost control
   c. Professional groups recognizing their accountability
   d. Regulatory agencies demanding cost-effectiveness
3. A comprehensive quality assurance evaluation includes the following:
   a. System evaluation of client treatment protocols and resource allocation
   b. Consumer evaluation of satisfactory meeting of client needs
   c. Clinical evaluation of outcomes of client care plan and optimum use of treatment process
4. Psychiatric and mental health nurses commonly function in clinical evaluation activities
   a. *Nursing audit* — designed to identify and examine the performance of specific aspects of nursing care, such as nursing process or a nursing procedure
   b. *Process audit* — used to compare particular nursing actions against established standards
   c. *Outcome audit* — designed to ascertain the desired client outcomes as they relate to the actual outcomes
5. All quality assurance programs use a common audit format (checklist with criteria for each care category) to ensure consistency
6. The JCAHO recommends the inclusion of seven components to develop an effective quality assurance program
   a. Identify the problem
   b. Set priorities for problem assessment and resolution
   c. Establish clinically valid criteria
   d. Select the assessment method
   e. Identify the causes of the problem

    f. Implement corrective action

    g. Evaluate the resolution of the problem

D. The scope of practice for a psychiatric and mental health nurse also includes psychiatric evaluation of clients who present themselves to the health care system

  1. Knowledge of human behavior, psychopathology, and psychotherapy equips the psychiatric and mental health nurse to perform the initial evaluation and then to arrange for care by other members of the mental health team

  2. The psychiatric evaluation determines a client's danger to self or others, ability to provide self-care, and degree of reality impairment

  3. It precisely describes the client's emotional and intellectual functioning at a specific time

  4. The evaluation is conducted during a private interview; the nurse listens attentively and observes the client closely

  5. A psychiatric evaluation has three components

    a. Identifying the presenting problem

      (1) Obtain the client's description of the presenting problem

      (2) Determine the problem's onset

      (3) Obtain the client's perception of the problem

      (4) Determine the client's perception of what caused the problem

    b. Taking a history

      (1) Medical

      (2) Family

      (3) Social

      (4) Psychiatric

      (5) Personal

    c. Performing a mental status examination

      (1) Note the client's appearance, reaction to the interview, and outward behavior

      (2) Note level of consciousness, short- and long-term memory recall, orientation, judgment, and intellectual functioning

      (3) Observe speech characteristics, thought patterns, and manner of communication

      (4) Observe affect for intensity and appropriateness

      (5) Note mood, looking especially for suicide or homicide ideation

      (6) Assess the client's insight and understanding of the problem

  6. Data are then organized and analyzed

  7. Medical and nursing diagnoses are made

  8. Development of a treatment plan completes the evaluation process

5 Theoretical models of behavior

I. Overview

A. Human behavior is best understood within a conceptual framework

B. A strong theoretical grounding provides the practitioner with an understanding of behavioral psychopathology and promotes thoughtful and logical practice

C. Nine models of human behavior are widely used; because human behavior is not fully understood, no model is considered right or wrong, better or worse than any other model

D. The practitioner's theoretical perspective will determine the conceptual model selected in developing a care plan

E. Psychiatric and mental health nurses commonly use an eclectic approach, drawing on several different theoretical models of behavior, to fashion practical and effective care plans

II. Psychoanalytic model

A. Sigmund Freud is considered the father of psychoanalytic theory

B. His theory states that deviations in human behavior result from unsuccessful task accomplishment during earlier developmental stages

C. Freud's psychoanalytic theory of behavior is built on five assumptions
   1. The personality consists of three structures: id, ego, and superego
      a. The *id* is present at birth
         (1) The id houses an individual's needs, drives, and wishes
         (2) Because the id always seeks immediate reduction from tension, it operates on the pleasure principle
         (3) The id is not oriented to reality
      b. The *ego* begins to form between ages 4 and 5 months
         (1) The ego develops because the id must negotiate with external reality to meet its needs
         (2) The ego mediates between the id and external reality
         (3) The ego operates in reality and can solve problems
         (4) To protect itself from being overwhelmed by anxiety, the ego uses defense mechanisms, such as repression
      c. The *superego* begins to develop at age 3
         (1) The superego is an outgrowth of the ego
         (2) It houses the conscience, one's inner sense of right and wrong

(3) Like the id, the superego is not reality oriented; it is concerned with the ideal and is rather rigid and moralistic in its application of what is right or wrong

2. Development occurs in five stages during which the child must master specific psychosexual conflicts to become a healthy, functioning adult; the names of the stages reflect the body area most associated with the child's source of gratification

   a. The *oral stage* occurs between birth and age 18 months
      (1) The child's needs are satisfied by oral gratification: feeding, exploring objects by placing them in the mouth, or exploring by using the lips
      (2) If needs are met, the child gains a feeling of trust and well-being
      (3) If needs are not met satisfactorily, the child becomes an adult who is afraid and ill-at-ease

   b. The *anal stage* occurs between ages 18 months and 3 years
      (1) The child develops an awareness of fullness in the rectum
      (2) The child takes pleasure in retaining or eliminating feces
      (3) If this stage is negotiated effectively, the child becomes an adult who can delay gratification to attain future goals
      (4) If this stage is inadequately negotiated, the child becomes an adult who is either excessively rigid and conservative or messy and destructive

   c. The *phallic (Oedipal) stage* occurs between ages 3 and 6
      (1) The child takes pleasure in exploring and manipulating genitalia
      (2) The child is attracted to the opposite-sex parent but realizes that he or she cannot sexually relate with this parent; the dilemma is resolved by identifying with the same-sex parent
      (3) During this stage, the superego develops and the conscience is formed
      (4) If needs are adequately met during this stage, the child develops a sex-appropriate identity
      (5) If needs are inadequately met during this stage, the child will become an adult whose sexual identity is confused and who has problems relating to authority figures

   d. The *latency stage* occurs between ages 6 and 12
      (1) The child has learned to express inner drives and urges in socially acceptable ways; sexual tension is sublimated into age-appropriate activities
      (2) If this stage is successfully negotiated, the child becomes an adult who can deal with various life situations
      (3) If this stage is not successfully negotiated, the child becomes an adult who has difficulty in developing social skills and who feels inferior to others

   e. The *genital stage* occurs between ages 13 and 20

(1) Corresponding with genital maturation is a reawakening of the sex drive

(2) The child expends energy establishing psychological independence from parents and family

(3) If this stage is completed successfully, an adult emerges whose personality structure is integrated, allowing the development of love and work relationships

(4) Unsuccessful completion of this stage results in an adult whose ability to establish intimacy and a strong personal identity is greatly compromised

3. Mental or psychological activity occurs on three levels

    a. The *conscious level* houses part of the ego

      (1) The conscious mind is much smaller than the unconscious mind

      (2) The conscious mind is reality based

      (3) Any mental information readily available to the individual is located in the conscious

    b. The *subconscious level* houses part of the ego

      (1) The subconscious acts as a filtering device between the external environment and the ego, and between the unconscious and the ego

      (2) Information stored in the subconscious can be called into conscious awareness

    c. The *unconscious level* houses the id and part of the superego

      (1) Comparatively, the unconscious mind is much larger than the conscious mind

      (2) The unconscious is not reality based

      (3) Information housed in the unconscious affects behavior; the information is unavailable to the conscious mind

4. Behavior is motivated by anxiety, the cornerstone of psychopathology

    a. Anxiety arises when unresolved conflicts are stimulated

      (1) To protect itself against overwhelming anxiety, the ego erects defense mechanisms

      (2) Deviant behavioral symptoms result from these defense mechanisms

    b. Severe anxiety may produce behavioral regression to an earlier developmental level

      (1) If regression occurs, the individual uses more primitive defense mechanisms

      (2) This compromises the individual's ability to function at an age-appropriate level

5. Behavior is always meaningful and often unconsciously motivated

D. The psychoanalytic model holds numerous implications for the nurse

  1. Understanding the psychosexual stages of childhood provides a framework for understanding behaviors observed in adult clients

2. Effective parenting can be promoted by teaching parents about the child's needs during each psychosexual stage

3. Successfully identifying manifestations of anxiety and the defense mechanisms used to control anxiety provides clues for planning nursing care

4. Defense mechanisms protect a client from overwhelming anxiety; the nurse should not deliberately interfere with them

5. All behavior is meaningful, often representing the unconscious needs and wishes of clients who do not always know why they behave as they do

III. Interpersonal models

A. Harry Stack Sullivan and Hildegard Peplau are two of the most prominent interpersonal theorists

B. Sullivan believed that human development results from interpersonal relationships and that behavior is motivated by the avoidance of anxiety and the attainment of satisfaction

1. He described three modes by which individuals relate to the external world

   a. The *prototaxic mode,* the most primitive mode, is used mainly by infants, who do not yet view themselves as differentiated individuals

   b. The *parataxic mode* is commonly used by children and juveniles, who view themselves as differentiated from the world but who do not clearly understand how they and the rest of the world fit together

   c. The *syntaxic mode,* the highest mode of relating, is used by older children and adults, who can understand complex situations and use consensual validation

2. Sullivan believed that the *self system* (akin to the ego in Freud's psychoanalytic model) is designed to protect one against anxiety and to allow one to obtain satisfaction; the self system has three components

   a. The "good me" makes approved behaviors a part of the self; self-identification is positive

   b. The "bad me" identifies disapproved behaviors that, if carried out, would be viewed as negative by the self

   c. The "not me" denies the existence of behaviors that, if identified with the self, would arouse intense anxiety

3. Sullivan outlined six stages of growth and development (see Chapter 3, Section IV, A2); within each stage, the individual possesses the tools for completing the developmental tasks central to any given stage

4. Sullivan's interpersonal model holds numerous implications for the nurse

   a. The nurse can strengthen the "good me" by assisting the client to develop positive behaviors

      b. Teaching clients how to use consensual validation assists them to function in the syntaxic mode

      c. If a client's world view is fragmented (parataxic mode), a corrective relationship with the nurse will promote the client's ability to relate to the world on an integrated (syntaxic mode) level

      d. Exploration of a behavior is not as important as exploration of the anxiety associated with that behavior

      e. The nurse can design corrective experiences aimed at reversing developmental deficiencies

C. Hildegard Peplau drew on Sullivan's theory to propose an interpersonal nursing theory that advanced the practice of psychiatric nursing by defining it as an interpersonal process

    1. She proposed that nurses must promote the nurse-client relationship to build trust and foster healthy behavior

    2. She demonstrated how nurses could use psychodynamic concepts and counseling techniques with clients

    3. Peplau maintained that the therapeutic use of self promotes healing

    4. Through examination of the nurse-client relationship, both nurse and client benefit from the therapeutic relationship

      a. The therapeutic relationship is directed toward meeting the client's needs and is thus client focused

      b. All nurses must examine their responses to clients, but they should never be the focus of the therapeutic relationship

      c. Consistency in the nurse-client relationship fosters the development of trust

      d. Nurses are accountable to clients for the quality of their work during the nurse-client therapeutic relationship

      e. The nurse-client relationship moves through four distinct phases

        (1) In the *orientation phase,* the nurse establishes the parameters of the relationship

        (2) In the *identification phase,* the client describes the problem

        (3) In the *exploitation phase,* the nurse and the client examine the problem within the context of the therapeutic relationship

        (4) In the *resolution phase,* the nurse and the client summarize progress made in resolving the problem and formally terminate the relationship

    5. Believing anxiety to be an important motivator of behavior, Peplau classified anxiety into four levels

      a. *Mild anxiety* is characterized by heightened alertness and enhanced problem-solving ability

      b. *Moderate anxiety* is characterized by occasional episodes of selective inattention, distraction, and impaired problem-solving ability

      c. *Severe anxiety* is characterized by a greatly reduced perceptual field, selective inattention, and markedly impaired problem-solving ability

        d. *Panic anxiety* is characterized by a perceptual field that has been narrowed to the object of anxiety, loss of ability to see environmental details, extreme deviant behavior, and loss of problem-solving ability

    6. Peplau's interpersonal model has the following nursing implications:

        a. The therapeutic relationship serves as a corrective experience that the client can use as a building block in developing other successful relationships

        b. The nurse employs empathy to access the client's feelings

        c. The nurse uses the self as a therapeutic tool to enhance the client's growth; a by-product is the nurse's personal growth

        d. Nursing is an interpersonal process in which the nurse and the client affect and are affected by each other

        e. Anxiety is interpersonally communicated

        f. Anxiety affects the client's ability to perceive a situation objectively and to generate alternatives

IV. Social model

    A. Gerald Caplan and Thomas Szasz, the prominent theorists of this model, postulate that the entire sociocultural environment influences mental health

    B. The social model embraces four fundamental principles

        1. Deviant human behavior is defined by the culture in which a person lives

            a. Szasz described the "myth" of mental illness, whereby a society labels someone considered undesirable as mentally ill

            b. This label, in effect, helps control undesirables by hospitalizing them

            c. Undesirable or abnormal behavior in one society may be considered normal in another society

        2. People can control whether they desire to conform to societal expectations

        3. Physical pathology defines illness and influences behavior but does not cause deviant behavior

        4. Crises precipitate deviant behavior because a person is vulnerable to sociocultural stress

    C. Caplan proposed that social conditions and interactions (family strife, poverty, inadequate education) dispose people to mental illness

    D. He applied primary, secondary, and tertiary health prevention principles to mental health

        1. Primary prevention involves avoiding disease

        2. Secondary prevention involves shortening a disease episode

        3. Tertiary prevention involves controlling the adverse impact of disease

    E. Nursing implications of the social model include the following:

1. The nurse collaborates with the client to change behavior
2. The client may accept or reject the plan to solve the problem
3. Therapeutic interventions are influenced by the sociocultural environment
4. The nurse has a moral obligation to provide mental health services that address all health prevention levels
5. The therapeutic approach involves using the entire social context of the client's life
6. Increased community involvement by the nurse enhances understanding of the client's environment

V. Existential model

A. This theory centers on an individual's present experiences rather than on past ones

B. Ludwig Binswanger, Frederick Perls, and William Glasser exerted much influence on existential theory

C. The existential model is based on four principles
   1. Alienation from the self causes deviant behavior
   2. The self imposes behavioral restrictions that cause the alienation
   3. Each person can make free choices about which behaviors to display
   4. People submit to others' demands rather than be themselves

D. Existential theory relies heavily on the assumption that people can make free choices from life's table of offerings

E. Nursing implications of the existential model include the following:
   1. The client has free choice of what is available in life
   2. The nurse works to help the client return from a state of self-alienation to a state of full life
   3. The nurse and the client are equals in humanity as they deal with the client's problem
   4. Human caring and a warm attitude help encourage the client to test different behaviors

VI. Nursing model

A. Several prominent theorists — including Martha Rogers, Dorothea Orem, Sister Callista Roy, and Hildegard Peplau — introduced models for nursing care that emphasized the person as a biopsychosocial being

B. This holistic approach draws on general systems, developmental, and interactive theories to promote nursing care characterized by collaboration between the client and the nurse

C. The nursing model focuses on caring (in contrast to other models, which focus on curing)

D. A central premise of the nursing model is that people live within a biopsychosocial framework that decides their health state

E. The nurse assesses a client's physical and emotional behavior, interprets the client's needs to others caring for the client, and changes the biopsychosocial framework to meet the client's needs

F. The nursing process is based on the holistic perspective of the nursing model

    1. Assessment (data collection) includes developing a health history of the client's physical or psychological problem

    2. Analyzing the data and formulating the nursing diagnoses require the nurse to consider all the physical, social, and emotional stressors that contributed to the deviant behavior

    3. Nursing care plans address all the client's needs in behavioral terms

    4. The nursing interventions implemented to achieve the nursing care goals fall under one of three categories

        a. Dependent actions follow a physician's order

        b. Independent actions provide individual, group, or family therapy

        c. Interdependent actions include referring specific areas of client need, such as psychological testing, to another mental health team member

    5. Evaluation of care is continuous and includes the client as an equal participant

G. The client's reactions to the nursing care given validate the nursing interventions

H. Nursing implications of the nursing model include the following:

    1. The client's needs direct the therapeutic relationship

    2. The nursing process is the basis for providing care

    3. Qualified psychiatric and mental health nurses provide individual and group psychotherapy

    4. The client's reaction to nursing interventions guides future interventions

    5. The nurse provides holistic care, using the services of other disciplines as needed

VII. Behavioral model

A. This theory proposes that all behavior, including mental illness, is learned

B. Unlike other theoretical models, which focus on the client's emotions, behavioral theory focuses on the client's actions

C. Behavioral theorists, such as Skinner, Wolpe, and Eysenck, believe that by focusing on the client's observed behavior, practitioners can use a strict scientific approach to study a therapy's effectiveness

D. Behavioral theory holds the following basic premises:

    1. There is no such thing as a defect in the personality structure

    2. Behavior that is rewarded will persist, whether the behavior is good or bad

    3. Unwanted behaviors can be eliminated through negative sanctions, such as punishment

4. Desired behaviors can be learned through positive sanctions, such as rewards

5. Diagnostic labels are irrelevant; the focus of treatment is the behavior that requires change

E. Behavior can be changed through behavior modification (see Chapter 10)

F. Nursing implications of the behavioral model include the following:

    1. People can learn to behave in socially desirable ways

    2. The behavioral approach can be used with different personality types

    3. Consistency is important; failure to adhere to the treatment plan guarantees failure

    4. The client's behavior (not pathology) is the focus of treatment

    5. Behavioral theory can be easily applied

VIII. Medical model

A. Disease is the cause of deviant behavior

B. The medical model focuses on diagnosis and treatment of the disease

C. Curing the disease restores normal behavior

D. Modern psychiatry is dominated by adherents to the medical model

E. Medical interventions to cure mental disease include the following:

    1. *Somatic therapy* — electroconvulsive and drug therapy

    2. *Interpersonal therapy* — psychoanalysis and psychotherapy

F. Therapists adjust treatment protocols based on the client's somatic response

G. Application of the medical model to mental illness has led to the identification of neurochemicals (such as enkephalins, serotonin, dopamine, and norepinephrine) as possible causes of deviant behavior

H. The medical model accepts socioenvironmental influences as potential causes of deviant behavior

    1. Social isolation, loneliness, and residence in an area associated with heavy drug use can cause a person to use drugs

    2. Working or living in an environment that exposes a person to high levels of carcinogens can cause disease

I. A central tenet of the medical model is the physician's control over the client's therapy

J. Clients are expected to admit their sickness, conform to a treatment plan, and get well

K. Nursing implications of the medical model include the following:

    1. The treatment of disease is based on the client's history and present condition, diagnosis, and laboratory studies

    2. The physician prescribes treatment and leads the treatment team

    3. Nurses and members of other health care disciplines are used in treatment when their expertise is required

    4. Interpersonal relations focus on the physician and the client

IX. Communication models

  A. Communication theory postulates that all human behavior is a form of communication

  B. The meaning of the behavior depends on the clarity of communication between sender and receiver

  C. Unclear communication produces anxiety, which results in behavioral deviation

  D. Three communication models are widely accepted

    1. Eric Berne's *transactional analysis* holds that communication is a unit called a transaction

      a. A transaction that is sent creates a complementary transaction when it is received and responded to by the receiver

      b. Communication occurs on three levels: parent, child, and adult

      c. When sender and receiver communicate on the same level, communication is referred to as a complementary transaction

      d. When transactions become crossed, the receiver responds differently than the sender expects, and communication disruptions develop

    2. Richard Bandler's and John Grindler's *neurolinguistic programming* focuses on word choices and on nonverbal communication

      a. People develop sensory channels (auditory, visual, kinesthetic) through which they receive communication

      b. Because they form a preference for one channel, communication harmony is established when both the sender and the receiver use the same channel

      c. Nonverbal communication (body language, speech pattern) is sent and received during any communication

    3. Paul Watzlawick's *pragmatics of communication* holds that behavioral deviation results from disrupted communication patterns (noncommunication, lack of congruency in communication, imperviousness, and punctuation discrepancies)

  E. Observing communication patterns can enhance understanding of behavioral disruptions

  F. Nursing implications of the communication model include the following:

    1. The communication pattern used with individuals, families, and social and work groups identifies the cause of behavioral deviation

    2. Improving communication improves behavior

    3. The nurse teaches the client effective communication techniques

    4. Effective communication by the client should be reinforced

    5. Eliminating behavioral deviation requires the client to participate in analyzing communication and in accepting responsibility for developing different communication styles

X. Humanistic model

A. Abraham Maslow was an American psychologist credited with founding humanistic psychology

B. Maslow is best known for describing a hierarchy of needs to understand human behavior

1. Physiologic survival

   a. Individuals at this most basic level are struggling for survival; working to obtain food, oxygen, rest, and maintaining physiologic stability, consumes their energies

   b. Individuals demonstrating behaviors that focus solely on these needs may have compromised health states

   c. If these basic needs go unmet, the individual could die; only partially meeting them causes personal discomfort

2. Safety, security, and self-preservation

   a. Satisfying these needs is important to provide structure, predictability, and protection to the individual's life

   b. If these needs are unmet, the person will experience separation anxiety and fear of self-harm

3. Love and belonging

   a. Being part of social groups and organizations allows a person to develop mutually fulfilling relationships

   b. The individual whose need for love and belonging is unmet will exhibit loneliness and experience feelings of alienation

4. Esteem and recognition

   a. The individual must feel like a worthwhile, contributing member of society; giving service to one's professional organization, serving on community boards, and appreciating one's own uniqueness are mechanisms for meeting this need

   b. If the need for esteem and recognition goes unfilled, feelings of inferiority and helplessness will result

5. Self-actualization

   a. To be self-actualized is to be self-fulfilled; people who know who they are, appreciate what they can do, face life's challenges confidently, have realistic expectations of self and others, and have a healthy sense of humor are self-actualized

   b. If self-actualization needs go unmet, the individual will experience loss of self-esteem and self-confidence

6. The aesthetic needs for truth, harmony, beauty, and spirituality

   a. Individuals who have become self-actualized will seek these needs

   b. Frustration of these needs can result in dissatisfaction and restlessness

C. Maslow believed it was important to study individuals who were well adjusted, not just individuals who were maladjusted

D. Maslow believed, unlike the behaviorists, that individuals were in control of their own behavioral choices, which were determined by underlying values rather than the external environment

E. Nursing implications of the humanistic model include the following:
1. Lower level needs must be met before higher level needs can emerge
2. Nurses must do a needs assessment, which enables them to determine appropriate intervention strategies for assisting clients to meet unmet needs
3. Individuals can choose to fulfill unmet needs but sometimes need assistance

6 Nursing research

I. Overview

A. Research is the systematic, logical, and empirical inquiry into the possible relationships among particular phenomena

B. It is a scientific method for gathering, analyzing, and disseminating new information

C. Nursing research is that scientific method applied to the study of any nursing problem, with the goal of expanding the theoretical basis of nursing through the discovery of new knowledge

D. Understanding the steps and techniques that researchers use enables the nurse to participate actively in research that benefits nursing

E. The nurse is then better able to judge the soundness of research findings before applying them in the clinical setting

F. All nurses are mandated by nursing practice standards (see Appendix A) to contribute to the growth of nursing knowledge by participating in the research process

G. Nursing research links nursing theory, education, and practice

H. Nursing theory is developed from practice and must be validated by research to be useful

I. Research can be descriptive, explanatory, or predictive

    1. *Descriptive research* obtains accurate information about the phenomenon under investigation; the investigator observes, describes, and classifies

    2. *Explanatory research* attempts to understand the relationship among the phenomena under investigation; the investigator explains observed events and their relationships to each other and to outside influences

    3. *Predictive research* uses statistical measures to forecast the relationships among phenomena

II. Types of nursing research

A. Nurses use several methods to identify, gather, and analyze information

B. The method selected depends on which questions the nurse-researcher wants to ask

C. The investigator uses two broad types of nursing research: quantitative and qualitative

    1. *Quantitative nursing research* involves the systematic collection of data in numerical format, under strict researcher control, and the analysis of that data in order to describe, explain, or predict a particular phenomena (for example, research that describes the views held by adolescents, parents, and school personnel toward adolescent suicide)

    2. *Qualitative nursing research* involves the systematic collection and analysis of subjective information (with attempts to minimize researcher-imposed control in the absence of statistical methodology) in order to understand the depth of a particular phenomena (for example, research that explores the experience of survival and bereavement after a loved one dies from acquired immunodeficiency syndrome [AIDS])

D. Because many of the research questions that interest nurses are complex, some researchers believe that neither the qualitative nor the quantitative method of research alone is sufficient

E. Increasing numbers of research studies are using both qualitative and quantitative methods (for example, a study of the psychological distress that can result from using a computer versus a pen and pencil)

III. Phases of nursing research

A. *Gathering data,* the first major phase of nursing research, requires eight essential steps

    1. Consider research ethics and the rights of human subjects

        a. Before gathering research data, the nurse must understand the risks and the benefits inherent in any research study

        b. Because most nursing research involves human subjects, the nurse must carefully consider the procedures used in order to protect the rights of those subjects

        c. Subjects have the right to refuse participation in the study, and those who volunteer have the right to sign an informed consent before research begins

        d. Subjects have the right to privacy, confidentiality, and fair treatment

        e. The American Nurses Association's "Human Rights Guidelines for Nurses in Clinical and Other Research" addresses research problems of particular concern to nurses

    2. Select a research problem

        a. A thorough research investigator spends considerable time selecting and defining a problem for study, because the problem is the foundation of and provides direction for the study

        b. Practical experience, scientific literature, and untested theory are all rich sources of research problems (for example, a nurse working with AIDS clients might want to examine what it is like to have the disease; another nurse, working with the same population, might want to explore whether nurses' attitudes toward AIDS clients influence the clients' emotional well-being

3. Identify the research question
    a. Although nurses may raise many legitimate questions about their practice, not all of these questions can be reasonably pursued through research
    b. Before selecting the research question, the nurse must consider four criteria
        (1) The research question should be of sufficient significance to nursing and health care
        (2) Researching the question should be feasible (inadequate time or funding, unavailability of subjects, lack of proper equipment, and ethical concerns are among the numerous problems that can hinder research)
        (3) Knowledge gained from the research must outweigh the cost of obtaining it
        (4) The topic should hold the researcher's interest over the duration of the study

4. State the research problem
    a. The problem must be worded clearly to guide the design of the study
    b. Experienced researchers differ as to whether the problem should be phrased as a statement or a question
    c. It must specify the subject to be studied, along with key variables amenable to observation or measurement
        (1) Variables are the properties that differ from one subject to another
        (2) Dependent variables are the concepts that the researcher wants to explain or predict; commonly referred to as "the consequence," they are assumed to vary with changes in the independent variables
        (3) Independent (or antecedent) variables presumably affect the dependent variables; the researcher typically manipulates these variables in an experimental study
        (4) Variables are not inherently dependent or independent (for example, alcoholism may be the dependent variable in a study of factors that predict alcoholism and an independent variable in a study of domestic violence)
        (5) Variables should be placed in a theoretical or conceptual context
    d. The scope of the problem must be precisely delineated so that the research direction is evident (for example, "What is the relationship between perception of autonomy and job satisfaction in a group of psychiatric nurses?" The independent variable [perception of autonomy] is presumed to affect the dependent

variable [job satisfaction] of a specific population [psychiatric nurses])

5. Review the literature

    a. All research studies demand a thorough review of the appropriate literature

    b. Timing of the review depends on the nature of the research question

        (1) In most quantitative studies, the researcher conducts a thorough review before collecting data to identify potential gaps in the literature and to examine the approaches others have taken in studying a particular problem

        (2) In qualitative studies, the researcher commonly collects data before an extensive review to minimize researcher bias

    c. The review must include data-based and conceptual literature

        (1) Data-based literature addresses the problem of interest

        (2) Conceptual literature addresses underlying theories of the problem

    d. The review should also encompass statistics, research findings, methods and procedures, opinions, beliefs, and clinical impressions and situations relevant to the study

    e. The review should include primary and secondary research sources

        (1) Primary sources are articles written by the investigator who conducted the research or proposed the theory

        (2) Secondary sources are reviews of primary sources; although they frequently prove useful in supplying additional references on the topic, secondary sources should not be substituted for primary sources because they provide less detail and may expose the researcher to the second author's bias

6. Develop a theory (theoretical framework)

    a. A theory is a statement that attempts to describe, explain, or predict some phenomenon

    b. It guides the researcher in separating critical and necessary factors or relationships from accidental ones

    c. A theory consists of the abstract concepts being studied (such as health, anxiety, stress, or pain) and a set of propositions that depict the relationships among the concepts

    d. A theory is built inductively from research and then tested deductively by research

        (1) Most qualitative research is inductive; researchers primarily use it to develop a theory

        (2) Most quantitative research is deductive; researchers primarily use it to test a theory

7. Develop a hypothesis

    a. After stating the problem, reviewing the literature, and choosing a theoretical framework, the researcher formulates a hypothesis

    b. The hypothesis is derived from the theory and serves as a prediction or preliminary explanation of the relationships among variables

    c. Written as a declarative statement, it delineates the relationship between at least two variables, one dependent and one independent

    d. A hypothesis can be simple or complex, formulated directionally or nondirectionally

       (1) A *simple hypothesis* expresses an expected relationship between one independent and one dependent variable (for example, "There is a relationship between perception of autonomy and job satisfaction among psychiatric nurses")

       (2) A *complex hypothesis* expresses a relationship between two or more independent variables and two or more dependent variables (for example, "A relationship exists between level of education, perception of autonomy, and job satisfaction among psychiatric nurses")

       (3) In a *directionally formulated hypothesis,* the researcher predicts the nature as well as the existence of a relationship (see the first example above)

       (4) In a *nondirectionally formulated hypothesis,* the researcher predicts the existence of a relationship only (for example, "Nurses with higher education who perceive more autonomy in their work will experience greater job satisfaction than nurses with less education who perceive their work as less autonomous")

    e. Hypotheses are classified as either research or statistical hypotheses

       (1) A research hypothesis expresses a relationship between the independent and the dependent variables (the examples above are research hypotheses)

       (2) Conversely, a statistical (or null) hypothesis states that no relationship exists between the independent and dependent variables

8. Build the research design

    a. The design is a framework that the researcher creates, a set of instructions that tell the researcher how to collect and analyze data in order to answer a specified research problem

    b. The problem statement, literature review, theory, and hypothesis all contribute to this design

B. *Manipulating data,* the second major phase of nursing research, involves measurement and analysis of quantitative and qualitative information

    1. In many quantitative studies, nurse researchers use instruments or tools to measure subjective psychosocial concepts (such as attitudes, stress, and social support systems) that cannot otherwise be measured

a. Before using any tool, the nurse must evaluate its validity and reliability
   (1) *Validity* is the extent to which an instrument measures what it
      claims to measure (for example, does a tool that claims to
      measure introversion or extroversion really measure those
      traits?)
   (2) There are three different types of validity: criterion, content,
      and construct
   (3) *Reliability* is the extent to which an instrument yields the
      same results on repeated trials
   (4) The researcher uses four methods — retest, split-half, alterna-
      tive form, and coefficient alpha — to evaluate an
      instrument's reliability

b. When manipulating quantitative data, the researcher uses statistical and sampling techniques to assign numerical values to
   what has been measured
   (1) *Statistical techniques* enable the researcher to analyze result-
      ing numerical values
      (a) Scales are commonly used to express all possible values
         of a given measurement
      (b) As an example, job satisfaction might be rated on a scale
         of 1 (least satisfied) to 6 (most satisfied)
   (2) *Sampling* is the process of selecting a portion of a population
      to represent the entire group
      (a) Probability sampling uses random selection, so that every
         member of the population has an equal chance of being
         selected
      (b) Commonly used probability methods include simple ran-
         dom, stratified random, cluster, and systematic sam-
         pling
      (c) Probability sampling, the basis of most statistical testing,
         avoids bias but can be costly and inconvenient
      (d) Nonprobability sampling uses arbitrary judgment or de-
         fined characteristics of the population as samples
      (e) Samples of convenience or selections by quota are exam-
         ples of nonprobability samples
      (f) The researcher should use as large a sample as possible,
         given the constraints of the study

c. Once the data have been collected in a quantitative study, researchers use statistical analysis to make sense out of the findings; the analysis can be descriptive or inferential
   (1) Descriptive statistics organize, summarize, and present infor-
      mation coherently (for instance, measurement of the mean,
      median, mode, and standard deviation of the sample)
   (2) Inferential statistics make inferences about populations based
      on the samples taken from them, using the logic that

chance is the only thing that produces variations in the study

    (a) Inferential statistics test the hypothesis

    (b) Examples of inferential statistical tests include t-tests, F tests, chi-square, ANOVA, and regression analysis

2. Qualitative research focuses on human subjectivity, using inductive reasoning, natural settings, descriptive data, and process-oriented questions; examples include case studies, grounded theory, phenomenology, and ethnography

    a. *Case studies* provide an in-depth examination of one or more subjects to develop a profile of what happens to individuals in a given situation

    b. *Grounded theory* is inductively derived from studying the phenomenon it represents

        (1) The research question in a grounded study identifies the phenomenon to be studied (for example, "How do nurse psychotherapists experience the termination phase of therapy?")

        (2) The research is a continual process of making comparisons and asking questions

        (3) Data are collected (usually by interview and field notes) and analyzed until the researcher reaches a saturation point

    c. *Phenomenology* explores the experience of life as it is lived (for example, "What is the experience of living with AIDS?"); analysis then focuses on abstracting the essential meaning of the experience

    d. *Ethnography* examines the norms, values, and knowledge of a specific culture (for example, "What does self-care mean in the culture of the intensive care unit?")

        (1) In this type of study, the researcher uses interviews, participant observations, and records to focus on the sample's culture rather than the individual experience

        (2) Data analysis proceeds concurrently with data collection

C. *Reporting data,* the final phase of nursing research, uses descriptive or inferential statistical methods to reveal the results of the study

    1. The final research report must identify the methods used to analyze data (such as the computer software used)

    2. The report may use inferential statistics to predict whether relationships in the study sample are likely to occur in the population at large

        a. A report that uses these statistics should also include information needed to assess the findings

        b. Such information includes the statistical test used (for example, t test, ANOVA), the magnitude of the test, the degrees of freedom, the probability level, and the direction of the effect found

3. The researcher should evaluate the results and interpret the implications according to the original hypothesis, including a statement that clearly expresses whether the results are statistically significant (that is, whether they do or do not support the hypothesis)

4. The report should clearly and thoroughly present the researcher's conclusions about the accuracy and meaning of the results

5. The report also should address the importance of the study, commenting on the applicability of findings to the general population, implications for nursing practice, and directions for future research

7 Therapeutic communication

I. Overview

A. Communication is the process by which people transmit ideas and feelings to one another

B. According to communication theory, behavior is a form of communication that is influenced by a person's culture and experiences

C. Communication can be verbal or nonverbal, constructive or destructive
   1. Verbal communication is the use of spoken or written language to transmit information; it includes how words and phrases are used to convey meaning
   2. Nonverbal communication is the use of physical movement to convey messages; besides body language, it also can include such disparate elements as voice sounds (groans or grunts to convey displeasure) and hair and clothing styles (to promote a certain image)
   3. Constructive communication from the sender confirms the receiver's importance and promotes self-esteem
   4. Destructive communication from the sender belittles the receiver's importance and diminishes self-esteem

D. Therapeutic communication is an interactive process that occurs between the client and the health professional; meaningful and intense, it focuses solely on the client's problems (see *Characteristics of social and therapeutic relationships*)
   1. Therapeutic communication is the foundation for establishing a therapeutic nurse-client relationship
   2. It requires the nurse to select words and phrases carefully in order to establish a dialogue with the client
   3. Its purpose is to elicit information about a client's needs, feelings, and ideas so the nurse can better understand the client's problems and develop interventions that strengthen a client's insight and self-control

II. Principles of therapeutic communication

A. Genuineness
   1. The nurse must display a sincere interest in the client and the client's problems

Characteristics of social and therapeutic relationships

In an effective nurse-client relationship, the psychiatric and mental health nurse uses therapeutic communication to shed light on and promote healthy changes in the client's behavior. The chart below contrasts important differences between a therapeutic relationship and a purely social one.

Social relationship	Therapeutic relationship
Focuses on mutual sharing, with each participant giving and taking	Focuses on the client, with the nurse giving and the client taking
Promotes mutual pleasure	Promotes client healing
Has no time constraints	Is time-limited
Does not involve a contract	Involves a contract between the nurse and the client
Does not require the participants to examine their behavior or to possess a specialized knowledge base	Requires the nurse to have a profound understanding of the nurse-client relationship and to examine each participant's behavior from a theoretical perspective

Adapted from Bininger, Carol J., et al. *American Nursing Review for NCLEX-RN,* 2nd ed. Springhouse, Pa.: Springhouse Corporation, 1992.

   2. Such authenticity conveys the message that the client can discuss anything with the nurse

B. Respect
   1. The nurse must have a positive regard for the client
   2. Nonjudgmental acceptance of the client's ideas and beliefs communicates the nurse's willingness to work with the client

C. Honesty
   1. A consistent, open, and frank approach promotes authenticity in the nurse-client relationship
   2. The client will be more likely to accept and trust a nurse who has nothing to hide

D. Concreteness
   1. The nurse should use clear, specific, concrete language rather than abstractions when communicating with the client
   2. Clear language focuses on specific areas that trouble the client and prevents misunderstandings by either party

E. Assistance
   1. The nurse must exhibit a willing commitment to the nurse-client relationship
   2. This conveys that the nurse has something of value to offer the client

    F. Protection

        1. The client must feel safe from confrontations with threatening forces (either self-harm or harm from others)

        2. Ensuring the client's safety promotes a successful relationship

    G. Permission

        1. Feeling free to explore new ways of dealing with past problems builds the client's autonomy

        2. Learning to try alternative behaviors is central to eliminating the client's problems

III. Blocks to constructive communication

    A. Giving advice prevents the client from forming independent conclusions and promotes dependence

    B. Providing false reassurance may inhibit the client from disclosing true feelings

    C. Asking too many "why" questions yields scant information and may overwhelm the client, leading to stress and withdrawal

    D. Using emotionally charged language may intimidate or shame the client and lead to withdrawal

    E. Straying from the client's agenda shifts the thrust of the nurse-client interaction away from the client's concerns; a client who detects the nurse's disinterest will feel unimportant and demeaned

    F. Using clichés shows a poor understanding of the client's uniqueness and conveys unwillingness to get involved, possibly leading the client to feel unheard, alone, discounted, and misunderstood

    G. Delivering double messages (such as contradicting a verbal message with a nonverbal one) confuses the client, who may become indecisive, anxious, and withdrawn

    H. Lecturing the client inhibits problem solving and suggests that the client is incapable of independent thinking

IV. Requirements for therapeutic communication

    A. Maintain privacy

        1. The client may be embarrassed or afraid to disclose personal and private information

        2. Fear that the conversation will be overheard by or revealed to others can discourage the client from being open and honest

    B. Preserve the client's self-esteem

        1. Conveying an unconditional and positive regard for the client promotes self-disclosure

        2. The client needs to feel valued and respected regardless of behavior or physical appearance

C. Choose words carefully
1. Language influences the therapeutic atmosphere
2. The nurse should avoid judgmental, demeaning, or threatening terms

D. Ask questions in a precise order
1. First, ask how the client would describe the situation or problem
   a. This question is emotionally neutral and elicits important data
   b. It immediately involves the client and conveys the nurse's interest
2. Next, ask what the client thinks about the situation or problem
   a. The client's thoughts provide assessment data
   b. Soliciting the client's interpretation maintains involvement
3. Finally, ask how the client feels about the situation or problem
   a. Sharing feelings may be frightening to the client, especially when the interview begins; covering this essential assessment step later in the interview commonly elicits useful information
   b. The nurse should accept and evaluate the client's feelings nonjudgmentally

V. Techniques of therapeutic communication

A. Listening
1. Focusing intently on the client enables the nurse to hear and analyze everything the client is saying
2. Such attention can alert the nurse to the client's communication patterns

B. Restating
1. Succinct rephrasing helps ensure the nurse's understanding and emphasizes important points in the client's message
2. It also confirms the nurse's attention, interest, and empathy and may promote further disclosure

C. Using broad openings
1. General statements or questions (such as "How's it going?") to initiate a conversation encourage the client to raise any subject
2. They also focus the discussion on the client and demonstrate the nurse's willingness to interact

D. Clarifying
1. Asking for clarification of a confusing or vague message demonstrates the nurse's desire to understand what the client is saying
2. It also can elicit more precise information crucial to the client's recovery

E. Confrontation
1. This technique calls attention to discrepancies in a client's communication patterns (for example, noting an apparent contradiction between verbal and nonverbal messages simultaneously communicated by the client)

      2. After confronting the client with the discrepancy, the nurse waits for a response

F. Focusing

      1. With this technique, the nurse assists the client in directing attention to something specific

      2. It fosters the client's self-control and helps avoid vague generalizations, thereby enabling the client to accept responsibility for facing problems

G. Silence

      1. Refraining from making comments can have several benefits: it gives the client time to talk, think, and gain insight into problems and permits the nurse to gather more information

      2. The nurse must use this technique judiciously, however, or else the client may perceive the nurse's silence as disinterest or rejection

H. Suggesting (presenting alternatives for the client to consider)

      1. Used during the working phase of the nurse-client relationship, this technique can help the client see previously untapped options

      2. When used correctly, the technique gives the client the opportunity to explore the pros and cons of numerous choices

      3. It must be used carefully to avoid directing the client

I. Sharing perceptions

      1. In this technique, the nurse attempts to describe the client's feelings and then seeks corrective feedback from the client

      2. This allows the client to clarify any misperceptions and gives the nurse a better understanding of the client's true feelings

VI. Guidelines for establishing therapeutic communication

A. Attend to the reality of the client's experience

      1. Focus on the client's questions and feelings

      2. Seek more data on the client's perceptions and thoughts

B. Give the client information

      1. Explain what to expect from the staff

      2. State the nursing unit's rules

      3. Describe what is expected of the client while on the unit

      4. Identify who will give care

C. Empower the client

      1. Include the client in care conferences

      2. Ask the client to contribute to care planning

      3. Determine the client's expectations

D. Anticipate the client's needs

      1. Begin discharge planning as soon as the client enters the therapeutic environment

      2. Provide privacy and personal space

      3. Conserve the client's energy to allow for healing

      4. Provide diversional activities as the client's energy level increases

E. Be accountable to the client

      1. Keep the client informed about the care plan

      2. Ask for the client's input about care

8 Legal aspects of nursing practice

I. Overview

    A. Safe psychiatric and mental health nursing practice requires a basic understanding of the federal and state laws and regulations that affect nursing practice

    B. State laws that affect psychiatric and mental health nursing practice vary from state to state

    C. Nurses practicing psychiatric and mental health nursing should familiarize themselves with the laws of the state in which they practice

II. Torts

    A. A tort is a civil wrong

    B. It is a violation of an individual's private rights that entitles the wronged individual to seek damages from the wrongdoer

    C. Two areas of tort liability have an impact on psychiatric and mental health nursing practice: negligence (unintentional torts) and intentional torts

        1. Negligence

            a. For a psychiatric client to recover damages for a claim against a nurse, four elements of nursing negligence must be present

                (1) The nurse must owe the client a duty of care

                (2) The nurse must breach the duty of care

                (3) The client must suffer damages

                (4) The nurse's breach of duty must be the cause of the client's damages

            b. Whether a psychiatric and mental health nurse owes a client a duty of care depends on whether a nurse-client relationship had been established

            c. A psychiatric and mental health nurse owes a client a duty to use that degree of knowledge and skill normally possessed by professional peers and to provide nursing services that meet accepted standards of psychiatric and mental health nursing practice

            d. A psychiatric and mental health nurse breaches the duty owed a client if the nursing care provided fails to meet the standards

                (1) A standard of care is generally measured by comparing the actions (or inactions) of the psychiatric and mental health

nurse with the actions (or inactions) of a reasonable and prudent psychiatric and mental health nurse functioning under the same or similar circumstances

(2) A standard of care can be derived from the following sources:

(a) The Nurse Practice Act and concomitant regulations of the state in which the psychiatric and mental health nurse practices

(b) "Code for Nurses with Interpretive Statements," by the American Nurses Association (ANA)

(c) The ANA's "Standards of Psychiatric and Mental Health Nursing Practice"

(d) "Consolidated Standards Manual for Child, Adolescent and Adult Psychiatric, Alcoholism and Drug Abuse Facilities," by the Joint Commission for Accreditation of Healthcare Organizations

(e) Professional journals, such as *Journal of Psychosocial Nursing and Mental Health Services,* the official journal of the American Psychiatric Nurses Association

(f) Experts in psychiatric and mental health nursing

e. An injured client may file a lawsuit against a psychiatric and mental health nurse to seek compensatory damages for pain, suffering, and economic losses (such as medical expenses and lost wages) resulting from the nurse's negligence

f. Common negligence allegations brought against psychiatric and mental health nurses include failure to monitor for changes in a client's condition, abandonment (leaving a client unattended), medication errors, negligent supervision of staff, and failure to ensure client safety

2. Intentional torts

a. Unlike negligent acts, which suggest unintended carelessness, intentional torts signify an intent to commit the act

b. Intentional torts also differ from negligence in that the client need not show proof of damages; the client may be entitled to punitive damages (in addition to compensatory damages), which serves to punish the wrongdoer

c. Common allegations against psychiatric and mental health nurses for committing intentional torts include the following:

(1) Invasion of privacy commonly arises in conjunction with treating a psychiatric client without obtaining informed consent

(2) False imprisonment commonly arises in conjunction with involuntary confinement and the use of restraints or seclusion

(3) Battery or assault charges usually involve physical contact with a client (or threats to do so) without the client's consent

(4) Breach of confidentiality

    d. Psychiatric and mental health nurses can prevent or limit claims of negligence and intentional torts in several ways

      (1) Provide safe nursing practice in accordance with the profession's standards of care (the best line of defense is prevention)

      (2) Ensure adequate documentation in the client's record

      (3) Understand the doctrine of assumption of risk: a client who refuses treatment knowing that the refusal could cause harm to self or others assumes the risk of harm, and the nurse cannot be held liable for the client's refusal

      (4) Understand the doctrine of comparative negligence

        (a) If a nurse and a client are both found negligent, the damages the client seeks to recover from the nurse may be reduced

        (b) If the nurse's employer or another health care provider is found negligent along with the nurse, the employer or other health care provider must pay a portion of the damages

      (5) Become familiar with governmental immunity statutes, which may prohibit a client from suing a psychiatric and mental health nurse employed by a state or federal agency or institution

III. Informed consent

    A. All psychiatric clients have the right to determine the treatment they will accept or reject

    B. This right is encompassed in the legal doctrine of informed consent, which requires the psychiatric client to be advised of the contemplated treatment plan

    C. Health care personnel are required to obtain the client's consent before treatment

    D. The doctrine of informed consent is derived from common law and constitutional law

      1. Common law

        a. Common law is based on prior judicial opinions

        b. It recognizes a client's right to self-determination, the right to determine what shall be done to one's body

      2. Constitutional law

        a. The United States and individual state constitutions guarantee people certain fundamental rights; among them is the right of privacy

        b. Courts have interpreted the constitutional right of privacy to include the right to accept or reject medical treatment

    E. The right to informed consent is not an exclusive right; it must be balanced against certain state interests

   1. Each state has an interest in preserving life, preventing suicide, and protecting innocent third parties
   2. If a psychiatric client threatens self-harm or harm to others, a state's interest in preventing such actions could outweigh the client's right to refuse treatment
   3. The client would then be compelled to undergo treatment despite a personal unwillingness

F. Certain information must be disclosed to a psychiatric client in order to obtain informed consent
   1. The proposed treatment
   2. The material risks associated with the proposed treatment
   3. Alternative treatments available
   4. The material risks associated with the alternative treatments
   5. The consequences if treatment is not rendered

G. Different states have different legal standards to determine whether informed consent was appropriately obtained
   1. Most states have adopted the "prudent patient" standard, which requires health care personnel to disclose the information a reasonable or prudent client would need to know to give informed consent
   2. Some states subscribe to the professional standard, which requires health care personnel to disclose information that other reasonable and prudent health care personnel normally disclose to a client to obtain informed consent
   3. The more stringent prudent patient standard is in keeping with the trends of expanding clients' rights and including clients in the health care decision-making process

H. Problems with obtaining adequate informed consent can arise in various circumstances in psychiatric settings
   1. Generally, minors cannot give informed consent because they have not attained the age of legal capacity (18 in most states)
      a. The child's parent or legal guardian must provide the necessary consent
      b. Some state statutes contain exceptions that allow minors to give informed consent under certain circumstances (for example, if the minor is married or pregnant or is seeking treatment for drug use or drug dependency)
   2. An adult must have the capacity to make decisions in order to give informed consent
      a. Although an adult is presumed competent until proven incompetent in a court of law, a psychiatric client may be presented for treatment whose mental competency is questionable
      b. Most state statutes provide procedures for these occasions, requiring a court hearing to determine whether a client is competent and appointing a legal guardian, if necessary

  c. If a client is deemed incompetent, informed consent must be obtained from a legal guardian

 3. The doctrine of informed consent also applies to clients who are committed either voluntarily or involuntarily to a mental health facility

 4. Commitment, whether voluntary or involuntary, does not mean that a client is incompetent or that any rights have been forfeited

I. Certain exceptions permit psychiatric treatment without obtaining informed consent from a client

 1. In an emergency (for example, if a psychiatric client is found unconscious), consent to treatment will be implied

 2. Informed consent is not needed if disclosure of the information necessary to obtain the consent would adversely affect the client

J. The psychiatric and mental health nurse's role can vary in practice situations requiring informed consent

 1. Generally, obtaining a client's informed consent is the responsibility of the attending physician; the nurse commonly serves as a witness to the client's signature on a consent form

 2. If the nurse has reason to believe that the client was not adequately informed or may lack the capacity to give informed consent, the nurse should not permit the client to sign the consent form; instead, the nurse should provide adequate information or contact the client's guardian

 3. In some situations, the psychiatric and mental health nurse may be required to obtain informed consent for nursing procedures, or a nurse may be required to carry out a physician's order that the client is resisting; providing treatment that has been refused could expose the nurse to a lawsuit for invasion of privacy and for assault and battery

 4. Even if informed consent was previously obtained, the client may revoke it at any time

IV. Confinement

A. The psychiatric client may be voluntarily admitted or involuntarily committed to a psychiatric facility

 1. Voluntary admission is generally available to mentally ill adults whose mental health needs cannot be met without in-facility care or whose mental illness causes them to be dangerous to themselves, others, or property

  a. A client is deemed dangerous if he or she has threatened or attempted suicide, is substantially likely to harm another, is unable to provide basic needs to such an extent that serious bodily harm will ensue, or is substantially likely to cause serious damage to property

  b. A client who is voluntarily admitted has the right to be discharged under certain conditions (most states accept the following conditions; the nurse should consult applicable state laws before implementing voluntary discharge)

(1) The request must be documented in the client's chart

(2) The client must be discharged unless the facility seeks involuntary commitment (because the client poses a danger to self, others, or property) and obtains a temporary court order to retain the client pending a full hearing by a court

(3) If a temporary court order to hold the client is not obtained within 2 days of the request to be discharged, the client must be discharged

2. Involuntary commitment is required when a mentally ill adult is unwilling to be admitted voluntarily for treatment

   a. Specific statutory procedures must be followed to consummate involuntary commitment

   b. The determination permitting the involuntary commitment must be reviewed periodically

   c. Any mentally ill adult who is believed to need commitment will be assessed by a designated local mental health screening facility

   d. The client can come alone, be referred by a family member, or be brought to the facility by a law enforcement officer

   e. The client can be detained at the screening facility for 1 day for assessment and treatment

   f. Once the client is assessed by the screening facility, appropriate mental health services must be recommended for the client

   g. If involuntary commitment is deemed necessary by the mental health staff, the client will be committed to an appropriate facility as soon as possible, even if the client objects to the confinement

   h. If there is no need for admission or commitment, the client is referred to the appropriate clinic services

   i. A client cannot be committed involuntarily unless the client exhibits the same dangerous behavioral propensities exhibited by clients who seek voluntary admission

   j. The client may be confined involuntarily in an appropriate facility for up to 72 hours without a temporary court order; however, the facility must begin court proceedings for involuntary commitment soon after confinement

   k. The court must immediately review an application for a temporary court order authorizing retention of the client; if there is probable cause to believe that involuntary commitment is necessary, the court will issue the temporary order pending a final hearing

      (1) Probable cause means it is more probable than not that the client will be involuntarily committed after the final hearing

   (2) At this point, the client still has not been involuntarily committed

   (3) If the court finds that probable cause does not exist, the client must be discharged

  l. If probable cause is found to exist, a final hearing must be conducted within 20 days of admission; the client has the right to attend the final hearing and must be represented by counsel

  m. The court will authorize involuntary commitment if it finds clear and convincing evidence (beyond a reasonable doubt) of the need; if clear and convincing evidence does not exist, the client must be discharged

  n. Periodic court review and hearings for all involuntarily committed clients must be conducted 3, 9, and 12 months from the date of the first hearing, and annually thereafter

  o. If a psychiatric facility determines that a client no longer needs involuntary commitment, the client can be discharged pursuant to a statutorily required discharge plan

 3. The statutory procedures required for voluntary admission and involuntary commitment were designed to protect an individual's right to liberty, due process, and equal protection under the law

B. Seclusion or restraint of a psychiatric client may be needed under certain circumstances

 1. Seclusion and restraint are interventions used to protect a psychiatric client from the likelihood of injury to self or others; such interventions should not be considered punishment

  a. Restraint is usually accomplished through the application of such devices as cloth or leather wrist and ankle restraints

  b. Seclusion is usually accomplished by isolating a client in a locked room

 2. Numerous legal implications surround a determination to restrict a psychiatric client

  a. The doctrine of least restrictive treatment requires the use of restrictive measures only if necessary and only to the extent required to ensure the safety of the client and others; therefore, if a vest is adequate to restrain a client, a four-point restraint should not be used

  b. If a client is competent, informed consent must be obtained before seclusion or restraints are used

  c. If a client is incompetent, or a minor, consent must be obtained from the client's legal guardian or parent; the emergency exception to the requirement to obtain informed consent applies

  d. If a client suddenly becomes violent and is in imminent danger of self-harm or causing harm to others, action can be taken without the client's consent

e. Many state laws limit the use of seclusion and restraint to occasions when the client has attempted injury to self or others or has caused significant property damage

f. Many facilities have specific policies and procedures for using seclusion and restraint

g. Nurses should be thoroughly familiar with their state's statutes and with their facility's policies and procedures

h. Failure to use restrictive measures when indicated could expose a nurse to claims for injury to the client or a third party, such as another client or staff member

3. Once seclusion or restraints have been implemented, additional legal issues arise

a. An inappropriate decision to restrain or isolate a client could expose a nurse to potential allegations of assault, battery, and false imprisonment; explicit documentation of the client's behavior, the reason for the restriction, and justification for the type of restriction used are necessary

b. Close observation of the secluded or restrained client is vitally important, and the extent of the observation should be documented

c. State statutes and health facility policies and procedures address the requirements for a physician's order, its renewal, the length of time a client may remain secluded or restrained, the need for observation, and the maintenance of the client's hygiene

d. The psychiatric and mental health nurse must be familiar with these requirements and adhere to them

V. Assault and battery

A. Assault is an attempt or threat to unlawfully touch or injure another person; apprehension resulting from the potential contact is what gives rise to claims of assault

B. Battery is the unlawful and intentional touching of another

C. Assault and battery are intentional torts

D. Claims of assault or battery can arise in the psychiatric setting when:

1. The client assaults or batters another client, a staff member, or a third party

2. The client assaults or batters the nurse

3. A staff member assaults or batters a client or is accused of having done so

E. The psychiatric and mental health nurse must attempt to prevent these situations from happening and know the steps to take if an assault or battery situation arises

1. Professional literature has identified client profiles and situations that lead to assault and battery by clients

    a. The nurse should evaluate each client for the potential to engage in assault and battery

       (1) Has the client previously assaulted or battered anyone?

       (2) Is the client taking a medication, such as fluoxetine (Prozac), that is associated with client violence?

    b. After identifying a client's predisposition to assault and battery, the nurse should institute close observation and preventive interventions and document these measures in the client's medical record

    c. Situations that may precipitate client violence include:

       (1) Involuntary confinement

       (2) Invasion of a client's personal space

       (3) Limiting a client's behavior

       (4) Staff attitude toward a client

    d. Nurses should intervene to help a client to cope with these events and conduct staff teaching on appropriate attitudes

    e. If a nurse fails to act reasonably to prevent a client from assaulting or battering a third party, the nurse could be found liable for the third party's injuries

2. Staff abuse of clients does occur; a psychiatric and mental health nurse who has reason to believe that a staff member is abusing a client should report the suspicion to a supervisor or begin an appropriate investigation

3. Each health care facility should have policies and procedures that address these situations

4. Clients have brought claims of assault and battery against psychiatric and mental health nurses for implementing seclusion and restraint and for administering treatments, including forced medication, without the client's consent

VI. Client rights

  A. Psychiatric clients are entitled to the same rights that other clients enjoy

    1. A psychiatric client may not be deprived of any constitutional or common law right simply because of receiving psychiatric treatment

    2. In some instances, psychiatric clients are granted special legal protection because of their vulnerable status

  B. Basic client rights include:

    1. The right to receive quality health care

    2. The right to informed consent and informed refusal

    3. The right to privacy

    4. The right to have medical information treated in a confidential manner

    5. The right to obtain a copy of one's medical records, unless medically inadvisable

6. The right to receive treatment without discrimination because of race, age, sex, religion, ethnicity, or inability to pay

7. The right to maintain one's dignity

C. Many state laws contain specific requirements to protect the rights of psychiatric clients

    1. A psychiatric client's rights are violated if the client is:

      a. Presumed to be incompetent merely because of being mentally ill

      b. Using unnecessary or excessive medication as a punishment, for the convenience of staff, or as a substitute for treatment

      c. Subjected to experimental treatment, electroconvulsive treatment, psychosurgery, or sterilization without informed consent or judicial authorization

        (1) A competent client must be given the right to consult an attorney or anyone else and must give express written consent for such treatment

        (2) If the client is incompetent, a court hearing must be held with the client present and represented by counsel, and the treatment must be judicially authorized before it can be rendered

      d. Restrained or secluded unless such restraint or seclusion is legally permitted

      e. Subjected to corporal punishment

    2. Specific psychiatric client rights include:

      a. The right to the least restrictive treatment

      b. The right to have one's own clothing, limited personal possessions, and a place to store them

      c. The right to receive visitors, make phone calls, and write letters

    3. Many state laws require that a psychiatric client's rights be posted, given, or recited to the client on admission or shortly thereafter

D. Psychiatric clients have the right to privileged communication and confidentiality

    1. Communications between a psychiatric client and the health care provider are legally protected as privileged communications by state law; this means that information about the client must be kept confidential unless the privilege is waived by the client or some exception to nondisclosure exists

      a. Privileged communication statutes differ from state to state

      b. Most states do not specifically include nurses in the category of health care providers subject to a privileged communication statute

      c. If information disclosed to the nurse is necessary for treatment of the client, the information may be considered privileged; however, some courts will require a nurse to disclose confidential information if a specific statutory privilege for nurse-client communication does not exist

2. Nurses are required to maintain a client's right to confidentiality, with some exceptions

    a. A nurse is required to report acts of child abuse; if a psychiatric client admits to committing such acts, the nurse must disclose this information to the appropriate authorities

    b. If a psychiatric client threatens to harm someone, the nurse may have the duty to warn the intended victim or take some other action to make the threat known to a supervisor or civil authority

3. Because of the sensitive nature of the information contained in a psychiatric client's records, the federal government and some states have enacted legislation that provides special confidentiality protection to clients receiving drug and alcohol abuse treatment and psychological treatment

4. If a nurse discloses confidential information about the client without the client's consent, a claim of invasion of privacy or breach of confidentiality may ensue

VII. Documentation of care

A. Although mental health records are primarily maintained to foster communication among health care providers and thereby facilitate delivery of appropriate care, they also serve certain legal purposes

1. Mental health records are used as evidence in competency hearings and involuntary commitment hearings

2. They are also used as evidence in lawsuits when a client claims a health care provider has acted negligently or committed an intentional tort

3. Although mental health records are considered confidential, their contents may be disclosed during any legal proceeding so long as the information is reasonably related to the matter undergoing judicial review

B. A client's mental health records, whether manual or computerized, must be properly protected to prevent access by unauthorized individuals

1. Access to a client's mental health records must be limited to those health care providers who are involved in treating the client

2. A client's mental health records may be reviewed for the purposes of peer review, quality assurance, audits, and research; however, the confidentiality of the information gathered must be protected, and any report generated as a result of such reviews must not directly or indirectly identify the client

3. A client's mental health records or information derived from them should never be released to third parties, such as insurance companies, without the client's written authorization

C. Documentation appearing in the medical record should be objective, concise, and thorough; only pertinent information should be charted

1. Because the client has the legal right of access to treatment records, the psychiatric and mental health nurse should chart as if the client were reading the record
2. Documentation should reflect treatment rendered in accordance with prevailing standards of nursing care
   a. If the nurse's actions are subsequently questioned (for example, in a lawsuit), the nurse will be able to demonstrate that the correct standard of care was met
   b. Courts generally assume that treatment was not given unless it is documented in the client's record
   c. If a nurse testifies that certain treatment was rendered but it does not appear in the record, the nurse may not be believed, especially if the testimony is about an incident that occurred several years ago
3. A client's mental health record should never be altered to conceal a negligent act; a client's injury or an incorrect treatment should be charted without concluding who was at fault

9 Anxiety disorders

I. Overview

A. Anxiety is a subjective feeling of vague apprehension that an individual experiences in response to stress

B. Anxiety serves two primary purposes
1. It alerts the person to an actual or impending danger
2. It prepares the person to take defensive action (flight or fight)

C. Some forms of anxiety are normal; other forms may signal a medical or psychological problem or a primary disorder

D. Hildegarde Peplau classified anxiety by its intensity: mild, moderate, severe, or panic (for additional information on anxiety levels and appropriate nursing interventions, see *Levels of anxiety*)

E. More severe manifestations of anxiety can be dysfunctional, presenting in various syndromes characterized as anxiety disorders

F. The syndromes are marked by an underlying anxiety that the individual desperately tries to control

G. The psychiatric and mental health nurse can detect anxious behavior in a client by observing for certain physiologic, cognitive, and social-emotional responses (for additional information on these responses and corresponding nursing diagnoses, see *Responses to anxiety,* page 71)

II. Theoretical perspectives

A. Biological theory
1. Anxiety results from biochemical imbalances
2. Chemical imbalances cause the midbrain to release norepinephrine, which increases anxiety

B. Psychodynamic theory
1. Anxiety results from unresolved developmental conflicts (for additional information on developmental tasks and conflicts, see Chapter 3)
2. The ego erects defense mechanisms to protect itself from potentially overwhelming anxiety

Levels of anxiety

Hildegarde Peplau classified anxiety according to its level of intensity: mild, moderate, severe, or panic. The following chart presents the major characteristics of each anxiety level, along with appropriate nursing interventions.

ANXIETY LEVEL	CHARACTERISTICS	NURSING INTERVENTIONS
Mild	• Alertness • Optimum ability to solve problems and make independent decisions • Enhanced learning	• Support optimal functioning of the client.
Moderate	• Hyperalertness and vigilance • Impaired problem-solving ability (assistance needed) • Selective inattention • Complaints of feeling "uptight"	• Assist the client in talking through the experience and labelling accompanying feelings. • Show the connections between details. • Encourage the client to use appropriate relaxation exercises.
Severe	• Narrowed client focus • Severely impaired problem-solving skills • Inability to grasp meaning of communications, engage in self-directed activity, or make decisions • Numerous physiologic complaints • Dependence on others; demands for attention	• Provide the client with structure and direction. • Remain with the client, and provide constant attention until anxiety diminishes to a moderate level. • Administer medication as needed.
Panic	• Complete inability to solve problems • Possible feelings of suffocation or loss of contact with reality • Inability to recognize familiar people, objects, or situations, even when identified by someone else • Erratic behavior	• Establish a simple, nonstimulating, structured environment. • Remain with the client at all times. • Speak in quiet tones, and use touch cautiously. • Engage the client in large-muscle or structured activity that does not require the ability to concentrate or solve problems.

    C. Interpersonal theory

        1. Behavior is designed to attain security and satisfaction

        2. Anxiety results when expectations or needs are not met in interpersonal relationships

    D. Behavioral theory

        1. Anxiety is a learned response to stress

        2. Anxiety in a client can be effectively reduced by using various behavioral techniques

III. Generalized anxiety disorder (GAD)

A. Characteristics

    1. Excessive or unrealistic worry or apprehension about several aspects of the client's life

    2. Inordinate amount of energy expended on controlling anxious feelings

B. Criteria for medical diagnosis (see the *DSM-III-R* diagnostic criteria for generalized anxiety disorder on page 75)

C. Possible nursing diagnoses

    1. Anxiety related to feelings of helplessness

    2. Fatigue related to insomnia

    3. Sleep pattern disturbance related to inability to relax

    4. Altered health maintenance related to inattention to activities of daily living

    5. Impaired social interaction related to withdrawal from social contacts

D. Treatment

    1. Relaxation training (the most effective treatment approach in managing GAD)

    2. Benzodiazepine therapy during the early phase of treatment (optional)

    3. Psychotherapy in conjunction with relaxation training (optional)

E. General nursing interventions

    1. Assist the client in identifying events that tend to increase anxiety and those during which the client experiences relative internal calm

    2. Engage in anticipatory planning with the client

    3. Teach and practice relaxation techniques with the client

    4. Help the client work on one problem area at a time

    5. Accompany the client to activities that the client is too anxious to attend alone

IV. Panic disorder

A. Characteristics

    1. Episodes of extreme panic that can last from a few minutes up to a few hours

    2. Relatively anxiety-free periods between attacks of panic-level anxiety (unlike with GAD)

    3. Fear of future attacks because the episodes are unpredictable and the individual feels out of control during them

    4. Attempts by the client to impose severe limitations on life-style in order to stave off future attacks

    5. Possible development of phobias as the client tries to avoid anything associated with panic attacks

Responses to anxiety

Individuals respond to anxiety in various ways. Some of these responses are normal; others may signal a serious health problem. A client with an anxiety disorder, for example, typically exhibits many of the physical, cognitive, and social-emotional responses to anxiety listed below. These signs and symptoms can assist the nurse in formulating nursing diagnoses appropriate for the client's condition.

RESPONSES	NURSING DIAGNOSES
Physical	
• Restlessness	• Fatigue
• Tremulousness	• Pain
• Increased pulse and respirations	• Sensory-perceptual alteration
• Elevated blood pressure	• Sleep pattern disturbance
• Tightness in chest, neck, or back	• Altered patterns in urinary elimination
• Breathing difficulty	• Ineffective breathing pattern
• Perspiration	• Constipation
• Insomnia	• Diarrhea
• Headache	
• Nausea	
• Dizziness	
• Fatigue	
• Urinary urgency, frequency, or both	
• Constipation or diarrhea	
Cognitive	
• Inattentiveness, distractibility	• Impaired verbal communication
• Poor concentration	• Altered thought processes
• Forgetfulness	
• Blocking of thoughts	
• Rumination	
• Preoccupation, such as with body functions	
• Decreased ability to solve problems	
Social-emotional	
• Vague feeling of discomfort	• Anxiety
• Apprehension	• Fear
• Worry	• Altered parenting
• Expectation of danger	• Altered role performance
• Irritability	• Social isolation
• Lack of self-confidence	• Spiritual distress
• Tendency to cry easily	• High risk for self-directed violence
• Social withdrawal	• Altered nutrition
• Inappropriate responses to a social situation	• Altered sexuality patterns

B. Criteria for medical diagnosis (see the *DSM-III-R* diagnostic criteria for panic disorder on page 76)

C. Possible nursing diagnoses
   1. Anxiety related to extreme, unrealistic fear
   2. High risk for injury related to feeling of terror
   3. Ineffective individual coping related to apprehension and helplessness
   4. Impaired social interaction related to inability to differentiate harmful situations from safe ones

D. Treatment
   1. Benzodiazepine or antidepressant therapy
   2. Relaxation techniques
   3. Aerobic exercise (only after careful evaluation; some clients have experienced panic attacks from lactic acid buildup after exercise)

E. General nursing interventions
   1. Remain with the client during a panic attack
   2. Provide for safety needs to counter the client's impaired perception
   3. Administer medication as needed
   4. Assist the client in seeking a pattern to the attacks (for example, after vigorous exercise, during certain times of the day, at specific places or events)

V. Obsessive-compulsive disorder

A. Characteristics
   1. Intrusive, persistent, delusional, or destructive thoughts (obsessions) that the client does not want but cannot ignore
   2. Irrational, repetitive, ritualistic behaviors (compulsions) that the client uses in attempts to control the anxiety resulting from obsessions
   3. Inability to control the thoughts and behaviors, despite recognition by the client of their absurdity and intensity
   4. Marked interference with normal daily routines, consuming hours of the client's day
   5. Possible benefits (secondary gains) that the client experiences, thereby perpetuating the obsessive-compulsive behavior

B. Criteria for medical diagnosis (see the *DSM-III-R* diagnostic criteria for obsessive-compulsive disorder on pages 76 and 77)

C. Possible nursing diagnoses
   1. Anxiety related to feelings that are unacceptable to the client
   2. High risk for self-directed violence related to compulsive behaviors, such as mutilation
   3. High risk for violence directed at others related to hostility or aggression

      4. Self-esteem disturbance related to unwanted obsessive thoughts

      5. Altered health maintenance related to disruptions in carrying out activities of daily living

      6. Impaired verbal communication related to reduced ability to express unwanted feelings

  D. Treatment

      1. Behavioral techniques

         a. Desensitization, or graded exposure (having the client gradually engage in anxiety-provoking activities or situations)

         b. Modeling of desired behavior (showing the client how to respond to bothersome stimuli)

         c. Response delay (having the client wait for increasingly longer intervals before engaging in ritualistic behaviors)

         d. Thought stopping (having the client willfully interrupt unwanted, anxiety-producing thoughts by engaging in a competing activity or by yelling "stop")

      2. Benzodiazepine therapy (to control underlying anxiety)

      3. Nonreinforcement of secondary gains

  E. General nursing interventions

      1. Provide time for the client to carry out rituals

      2. Do not interrupt a ritual once it has started; to do so could result in panic-level anxiety

      3. Assist the client with self-care, as needed

      4. Have the client keep a journal about the events surrounding obsessive-compulsive behaviors

VI. Simple phobia

  A. Characteristics

      1. Intense and unrealistic fear of an object, person, or event

      2. Willingness of the client to do anything to avoid the phobic object, person, or event, regardless of the consequences

      3. Inability of the client to overcome the fear, despite recognition by the client that the fear is absurd

      4. Extreme anxiety on encountering the phobic object, person, or event

  B. Criteria for medical diagnosis (see the *DSM-III-R* diagnostic criteria for simple phobia on page 77)

  C. Possible nursing diagnoses

      1. Fear related to an irrational feeling toward something harmless

      2. Powerlessness related to an inability to control the fear

      3. Social isolation related to self-protected avoidance

D. Treatment
  1. Behavioral techniques
    a. Social-skills training, especially effective in ameliorating *social phobia* (fear and avoidance of a particular social situation)
    b. Desensitization, effective in ameliorating simple phobia and agoraphobia (fear and avoidance of public places)
  2. Benzodiazepine therapy (may be used to manage panic attacks, especially in agoraphobia)

E. General nursing interventions
  1. Never force the client to contact the phobic object; such contact may precipitate a panic attack
  2. Instruct the client in the behavioral techniques prescribed by the treatment team
  3. Provide reassurance that the client will not be forced to confront the phobic situation
  4. Initially, adjust the environment to accommodate the client's phobia; as treatment progresses, adjustment will not be necessary

VII. Post-traumatic stress disorder (PTSD)

A. Characteristics
  1. Grieving-like behaviors that result from a major and severe trauma, such as rape, assault, accident, fire, war, or natural disaster
  2. Extreme anxiety or fear and a sense of powerlessness or helplessness
  3. Varying onset and intensity of symptoms
    a. Acute PTSD: within 6 months of the event
    b. Delayed PTSD: later than 6 months after the event
  4. Extreme anxiety generated by reexperiencing the event (may lead to bouts of depression, substance abuse, or suicide attempts)

B. Criteria for medical diagnosis (see the *DSM-III-R* diagnostic criteria for post-traumatic stress disorder on pages 77 and 78)

C. Possible nursing diagnoses
  1. Post-trauma response related to the traumatic experience
  2. High risk for self-directed violence related to anger and self-blame over the event
  3. Sleep pattern disturbance related to persistent dreams about the event
  4. Anxiety related to feelings of insecurity and being unsafe

D. Treatment
  1. Individualized therapy directed toward helping the client achieve cognitive mastery over the traumatic situation
  2. Benzodiazepine therapy (may be prescribed to manage uncontrollable anxiety)
  3. Antidepressant therapy (may be prescribed if depression is evident)

(Text continues on page 78.)

Diagnostic criteria for anxiety disorders

The following chart presents the *DSM-III-R* diagnostic criteria for the anxiety disorders discussed in this chapter.

Generalized anxiety disorder

A. The person experiences unrealistic or excessive anxiety and worry (apprehensive expectation) about two or more life circumstances (for example, worry about possible misfortune to one's child when the child is not in danger, coupled with worry about finances despite a sound financial status) for 6 months or longer, during which the person has been bothered more days than not by these concerns (in children and adolescents, this may take the form of anxiety and worry about academic, athletic, and social performance)

B. The focus of the anxiety and worry in criterion A is unrelated to another Axis I disorder; for example, the anxiety or worry is not about having a panic attack (as in panic disorder), being embarrassed in public (as in social phobia), being contaminated (as in obsessive-compulsive disorder), or gaining weight (as in anorexia nervosa)

C. The disturbance does not occur only during the course of a mood disorder or a psychotic disorder

D. At least 6 of the following 18 symptoms often accompany the anxiety (do not include symptoms present only during panic attacks)

Motor tension
   1. Trembling, twitching, or feeling shaky
   2. Muscle tension, aches, or soreness
   3. Restlessness
   4. Easy fatigability

Autonomic hyperactivity
   5. Shortness of breath or smothering sensations
   6. Palpitations or accelerated heart rate (tachycardia)
   7. Sweating or cold, clammy hands
   8. Dry mouth
   9. Dizziness or light-headedness
   10. Nausea, diarrhea, or other abdominal distress
   11. Flushes (hot flashes) or chills
   12. Frequent urination
   13. Difficulty in swallowing

Vigilance and scanning
   14. Feeling keyed up or on edge
   15. Exaggerated startle response
   16. Poor concentration
   17. Trouble falling asleep or staying asleep
   18. Irritability

E. It cannot be established that an organic factor (such as hyperthyroidism or caffeine intoxication) initiated and maintained the disturbance

(continued)

Diagnostic criteria for anxiety disorders *(continued)*

Panic disorder

A. At some time during the disturbance, one or more panic attacks (discrete periods of intense fear or discomfort) have occurred
   1. The attacks were unexpected (that is, they did not occur immediately before or on exposure to a situation that almost always caused anxiety)
   2. The attacks were not triggered by situations in which the person was the focus of others' attention

B. Either four attacks have occurred within 4 weeks, or, following at least one attack, fear of having another attack has persisted for at least 1 month

C. At least four of the following symptoms developed during at least one of the attacks
   1. Shortness of breath (dyspnea) or smothering sensations
   2. Dizziness, unsteady feelings, or light-headedness
   3. Palpitations or accelerated heart rate (tachycardia)
   4. Trembling or shaking
   5. Sweating
   6. Choking
   7. Nausea or abdominal distress
   8. Depersonalization or derealization
   9. Numbness or tingling sensations (paresthesia)
   10. Flushes (hot flashes) or chills
   11. Chest pain or discomfort
   12. Fear of dying
   13. Fear of going crazy or of doing something uncontrolled

Note: Panic attacks involve four or more symptoms; attacks involving fewer than four symptoms are limited symptom attacks

D. During at least some of the attacks, at least four of the above symptoms developed suddenly and increased in intensity within 10 minutes of noticing the first symptom

E. It cannot be established that an organic factor (such as hyperthyroidism or amphetamine or caffeine intoxication) initiated and maintained the disturbance

Note: Mitral valve prolapse may be an associated condition but does not preclude a diagnosis of panic disorder

Obsessive-compulsive disorder (obsessive-compulsive neurosis)

A. The person experiences either obsessions or compulsions
   1. Obsessions
      a. The person experiences recurrent and persistent ideas, thoughts, impulses, or images that are, at least initially, intrusive and senseless (for example, a parent's repeated impulses to kill a loved child or a religious person's recurrent blasphemous thoughts)
      b. The person attempts to ignore or suppress such thoughts or impulses or to neutralize them with some other thought or action

Diagnostic criteria for anxiety disorders *(continued)*

      c. The person recognizes that the obsessions are the product of his or her own mind, not imposed from without (as in thought disorder)

      d. The content of the obsession is unrelated to another Axis I disorder (for example, the ideas, thoughts, impulses, or images are not about food in the presence of an eating disorder, about drugs in the presence of a psychoactive substance use disorder, or guilty thoughts in the presence of a major depression

  2. Compulsions

      a. The person performs repetitive, purposeful, and intentional behavior in response to an obsession, according to certain rules or in a stereotypical fashion

      b. The behavior is designed to neutralize or prevent discomfort or a dreaded event or situation; however, either the activity is not connected in a realistic way with what it is designed to neutralize or prevent, or it is clearly excessive

      c. The individual recognizes that his or her behavior is excessive or unreasonable (this may not be true for young children; it may no longer be true for people whose obsessions have evolved into overvalued ideas)

B. The obsessions or compulsions cause marked distress, are time-consuming (take more than an hour a day), or significantly interfere with the person's normal routine, occupational functioning, or usual social activities or relationships with others

Simple phobia

A. The person experiences a persistent fear of a circumscribed stimulus (object or situation), and the fear is *not* among the following:

  1. Fear of having a panic attack (as in panic disorder)

  2. Fear of humiliation or embarrassment in certain social situations (as in social phobia)

  3. Fears that are part of panic disorder with agoraphobia

  4. Fears that are part of agoraphobia without history of panic disorder

B. During some phase of the disturbance, exposure to the specific phobic stimulus almost invariably provokes an immediate anxiety response

C. The person either avoids the object or situation or endures it with intense anxiety

D. The fear or the avoidant behavior significantly interferes with the person's normal routine or with usual social activities or relationships with others, or there is marked distress about having the fear

E. The person recognizes that his or her fear is excessive or unreasonable

F. The phobic stimulus is unrelated to the content of the obsessions of obsessive-compulsive disorder or the trauma of post-traumatic stress disorder

Post-traumatic stress disorder

A. The person experiences an event that is outside the range of usual human experience and that would markedly distress almost anyone (such as a serious threat to one's life or physical integrity; serious threat or harm to one's children, spouse, or other close relatives or friends; sudden destruction of one's home or community; or the witnessing of another person being seriously injured or killed as the result of an accident or physical violence)

(continued)

Diagnostic criteria for anxiety disorders *(continued)*

B. The person persistently reexperiences the traumatic event in at least one of the following ways:
    1. Recurrent, intrusive, distressing recollections of the event (in young children, repetitive play in which themes or aspects of the trauma are expressed)
    2. Recurrent, distressing dreams of the event
    3. Sudden acting or feeling as if the traumatic event were recurring (includes a sense of reliving the experience, illusions, hallucinations, and dissociative, or flashback, episodes, even those that occur upon awakening or when intoxicated)
    4. Intense psychological distress at exposure to events that symbolize or resemble an aspect of the traumatic event, including anniversaries of the trauma

C. The individual persistently avoids stimuli associated with the trauma or exhibits a numbing of general responsiveness (not present before the trauma), as indicated by at least three of the following:
    1. Efforts to avoid thoughts or feelings associated with the trauma
    2. Efforts to avoid activities or situations that arouse recollections of the trauma
    3. Inability to recall an important aspect of the trauma (psychogenic amnesia)
    4. Markedly diminished interest in significant activities (in young children, loss of recently acquired developmental skills, such as toilet training or language skills)
    5. Feeling of detachment or estrangement from others
    6. Restricted range of affect (such as an inability to have loving feelings)
    7. Sense of a foreshortened future (for example, when a child does not expect to have a career, get married, have children, or live a long life)

D. The individual has persistent symptoms of increased arousal (not present before the trauma). as indicated by at least two of the following:
    1. Difficulty falling asleep or staying asleep
    2. Irritability or outbursts of anger
    3. Difficulty concentrating
    4. Hypervigilance
    5. Exaggerated startle response
    6. Physiologic reactivity upon exposure to events that symbolize or resemble an aspect of the traumatic event (for instance, a woman who was raped in an elevator may break out in a sweat when entering an elevator)

E. Symptoms (criteria B, C, and D) last at least 1 month

Note: Specify delayed onset if symptoms do not appear for at least 6 months after the trauma

Source: *Diagnostic and Statistical Manual of Mental Disorders,* Third Edition-Revised. Washington, D.C.: American Psychiatric Association, 1987. Adapted with permission.

    E. General nursing interventions
        1. Encourage the client to recall the traumatic event; remain nonjudgmental and accept what the client is saying
        2. Provide a secure environment for the client to promote a sense of safety
        3. Remain with the client, especially one who is extremely anxious; reexperiencing the traumatic event can trigger severe or panic anxiety

4. Institute suicide precautions if the client manifests suicidal tendencies
5. Facilitate grieving by encouraging the client to express emotions generated from the event
6. Teach the client and family about post-traumatic behavior, and refer
them to support groups for additional help

Clinical situation

You are employed in a community mental health center. One of your new clients is Paul Smith, a 38-year-old accountant who says that he worries excessively about making mistakes. In fact, he is so preoccupied with doing things
correctly that he has been unable to function efficiently at work.

At home, Paul directs his energies toward making sure the family's finances
are in order and checking up on the activities of his wife and children. He also
worries about how neighbors and friends perceive him.

Paul tells you that he is exhausted from inadequate sleep and that he has experienced heartburn almost daily for the past several weeks. He describes himself as a worrywart, saying that he's always been a nervous person who is easily
upset when unforeseen things happen. He confesses that the quality of his life is
poor and that he is willing to do whatever it takes to stop worrying so much.

Assessment *(nursing behaviors and rationales)*

1. Perform a health assessment, especially inquiring about any changes in
Paul's appetite, sleeping, digestion, elimination, and cardiac functioning. *Anxiety causes changes in physiologic processes. Any deterioration in physical
health will need attention, and any physiologic cause for physical manifestations must be ruled out.*

2. Conduct a psychosocial assessment, especially inquiring about changes in
Paul's coping patterns, social supports, financial status, occupational stressors,
and interactional patterns. *A psychosocial assessment will assist in determining
the severity of impairment resulting from anxiety and factors associated with
anxiety.*

3. Assess Paul's perception of the current situation. *When planning and deliver-
ing appropriate care, the nurse must consider the client's perceptions. Until the
nurse can determine how the client views the current situation, generating a
plan of care specific to this client will be impossible.*

4. Assess Paul's ability to solve problems. *Such an assessment will help the
nurse determine the client's anxiety level. A particularly anxious client will not
be able to solve problems independently.*

Nursing diagnoses

• Anxiety related to the client's need to be perfect
• Fatigue related to the client's inability to sleep restfully at night and to feel re-
laxed during the day
• Altered role performance related to excessive worrying about doing every-
thing well
• Pain related to gastric reflux

Planning and goals

• Paul Smith will learn to manage anxiety so that role performance is unaffected.
• He will learn to relax during the day and to sleep more restfully at night.
• He will no longer experience discomfort from gastric reflux.

Implementation (*nursing behaviors and rationales*)

1. Involve Paul in a physical and psychosocial assessment. *This activity not only provides valuable baseline data but also communicates concern about the client's well-being and the conviction that the client is an active participant in his healing.*

2. Have Paul identify his most pressing problems. *Once the client has completed this exercise, he is in a position to determine which problem to tackle first. As he begins to deal with problems, he will feel empowered and, consequently, less anxious.*

3. Teach Paul how to engage in anticipatory planning rather than unproductive worrying. *Developing strategies in advance to manage potential problems will enhance the client's self-control.*

4. Engage Paul in cognitive exercises (for example, "What if...?" or "What would be the worst possible thing that could happen?"). *Learning to employ these cognitive techniques can help the client avoid the trap of automatically becoming anxious when he feels stressed or unsure about a situation. Instead, he will be able to develop a more objective perspective. Once the client learns to interrupt his automatic tendency to become anxious, he will be better able to manage his life.*

5. Teach Paul relaxation techniques to employ as soon as he becomes aware of feeling tense or nervous. *Like cognitive exercises, relaxation techniques will interrupt the client's automatic tendency to become anxious and will enhance his ability to maintain a balanced body chemistry.*

Evaluation

• Paul Smith uses a series of cognitive exercises and relaxation techniques in the morning before arising and during the day when he becomes aware of feeling tense.
• Paul sleeps restfully at night and reports having abundant energy throughout the day.
• Paul no longer experiences gastric reflux.
• Paul reports that he no longer feels a constant need to check up on family members and that his productivity level at work has increased markedly.

10 Addiction disorders

I. Overview

A. Addiction to psychoactive substances is a worldwide health problem

B. The mind-altering substances most commonly abused to the point of addiction are alcohol, narcotics, hallucinogens, and stimulants

C. Addiction (or chemical dependence, a term preferred by many health care professionals) is the end point of substance abuse; it is one of the most serious public health problems in the United States today

D. The symptoms and maladaptive behaviors associated with chemical dependence are categorized according to the addictive substance (see *Diagnoses for psychoactive substance disorders,* page 82)

E. Alcohol, by far the leading substance abused by Americans, is the principal focus of this section

F. Other drug addictions are reviewed in the context of their common effects on the body and the usual treatment approaches (see *Criteria for psychoactive substance dependence,* page 83)

II. Epidemiology of substance abuse

A. Alcohol

  1. About 67% of American adults consume alcohol; about 10% of them develop problems of dependence

  2. Roughly one-third of all hospital admissions are related to alcohol abuse

  3. The divorce rate for couples with an alcoholic spouse is seven times greater than that for other couples

  4. About 93% of high school students have tried alcohol by their senior year; about 6% of high school seniors consume alcohol daily

  5. Approximately one-half of all traffic accidents are alcohol related

B. Drugs

  1. Drug use is most prevalent among minority groups in metropolitan areas, but the problem crosses all racial, ethnic, socioeconomic, and geographic barriers

    a. About 10% of all Americans have tried cocaine, which is used most commonly by young adults aged 18 to 25

    b. About 3% of adults aged 18 to 25 have experimented with heroin

---

Diagnoses for psychoactive substance disorders

The following is a list of the *DSM-III-R* diagnoses for psychoactive substance disorders.
Alcohol Dependence
Alcohol Abuse
Amphetamine or Similarly Acting Sympathomimetic Dependence
Amphetamine or Similarly Acting Sympathomimetic Abuse
Cannabis Dependence
Cannabis Abuse
Cocaine Dependence
Cocaine Abuse
Hallucinogen Dependence
Hallucinogen Abuse
Inhalant Dependence
Inhalant Abuse
Nicotine Dependence
Opioid Dependence
Opioid Abuse
Phencyclidine (PCP) or Similarly Acting Arylcyclohexylamine Dependence
Phencyclidine (PCP) or Similarly Acting Arylcyclohexylamine Abuse
Sedative-Hypnotic or Anxiolytic Dependence
Sedative-Hypnotic or Anxiolytic Abuse
Polysubstance Dependence
Psychoactive Substance Dependence Not Otherwise Specified
Psychoactive Substance Abuse Not Otherwise Specified

Source: *Diagnostic and Statistical Manual of Mental Disorders,* Third Edition-Revised. Washington, D.C.: American Psychiatric Association, 1987. Reprinted with permission.

---

    c. About 3% of those aged 12 to 17 and 12% of those aged 18 to 25 have used lysergic acid diethylamide (LSD) or phencyclidine (PCP)

    d. Roughly 60% of young adults have experimented with marijuana or hashish, although recent governmental reports suggest that marijuana use by young Americans is declining

2. Narcotics abusers typically abuse more than one drug

    a. About 50% of abusers become chemically dependent

    b. Drug abuse afflicts about 6% of those taking sedatives, 8% of those taking antianxiety agents, and 9% of those taking amphetamines

3. One out of every two substance abusers meets the *DSM-III-R* diagnostic criteria for another mental illness, such as depression, schizophrenia, or borderline personality disorder

Criteria for psychoactive substance dependence

The following chart presents the *DSM-III-R* diagnostic criteria for psychoactive substance dependence.

A. At least three of the following criteria apply to the client:

1. Substance often taken in larger amounts or over a longer period than the person intended
2. Persistent desire or one or more unsuccessful efforts to cut down or control substance use
3. A great deal of time spent getting the substance, taking the substance, or recovering from its effects
4. Frequent intoxication or withdrawal symptoms when expected to fulfill major role obligations at work, school, or home (such as not going to work or school because of a hangover, going to work or school "high," being intoxicated while taking care of children), or substance use when it poses obvious physical hazards (such as driving while intoxicated)
5. Important social, occupational, or recreational activities given up or reduced because of substance use
6. Continued substance use despite knowledge of having a persistent or recurrent social, psychological, or physical problem that is caused or exacerbated by using the substance (such as continued heroin use despite family arguments about it, cocaine-induced depression, or continued drinking despite having an ulcer)
7. Marked tolerance (the need for markedly increased amounts of the substance [at least 50% increase] in order to achieve intoxication or desired effect, or markedly diminished effect with continued use of the same amount)

   Note: The following two items may not apply to cannabis, hallucinogens, or phencyclidine (PCP):

8. Characteristic withdrawal symptoms
9. Substance often taken to relieve or avoid withdrawal symptoms

B. Some symptoms of the disturbance have persisted for at least 1 month or have occurred repeatedly over a longer period.

Criteria for severity of psychoactive substance dependence

Mild: Few, if any, symptoms in excess of those required to make the diagnosis, and the symptoms result in no more than mild impairment in occupational functioning or in usual social activities or relationships with others

Moderate: Symptoms of functional impairment between Mild and Severe

Severe: Many symptoms in excess of those required to make the diagnosis, and the symptoms markedly interfere with occupational functioning or with usual social activities or relationships with others (Because of the availability of cigarettes and other nicotine-containing substances and the absence of a clinically significant nicotine intoxication syndrome, impairment in occupational or social functioning is not necessary for a rating of severe nicotine dependence.)

In Partial Remission: During the past 6 months, some use of the substance and some symptoms of dependence

In Full Remission: During the past 6 months, either no use of the substance or some use of the substance with no symptoms of dependence

Source: *Diagnostic and Statistical Manual of Mental Disorders,* Third Edition-Revised. Washington, D.C.: American Psychiatric Association, 1987. Adapted with permission.

III. Theoretical perspectives

A. Biological theory

1. Especially among those who abuse alcohol, a strong family history of abuse exists, suggesting a genetic link

2. Recent studies have shown evidence of brain chemistry alteration among substance abusers

a. A deficiency in dopamine and norepinephrine is apparent in cocaine abusers

b. A deficiency in enkephalins and endorphins has been noted in narcotics abusers and alcohol abusers

B. Psychological theory

1. Many substance abusers are attempting to lift underlying depression or to reduce tension, frustration, and psychic pain

2. Individuals with low self-esteem briefly feel empowered after using the substance

3. For some abusers, the substance relieves loneliness resulting from lack of meaningful relationships

C. Sociocultural theory

1. Many individuals become addicted during adolescence, when peer pressure is particularly strong

2. Substance abuse is directly linked to low socioeconomic status and racial oppression, as evidenced by high rates of abuse among Native Americans and poor Black males

3. Cultural beliefs about the responsible use of alcohol mitigate against abuse, as evidenced by the low rate of abuse among Jewish people

4. Social expectations and encouragement of consumption promote irresponsible use, as evidenced by the high rate of abuse among sociocultural groups that tolerate alcohol or drug consumption

D. Behavioral-cognitive theory

1. The addicted individual associates certain cues (such as the end of a work day or a weekend party) with ingestion of the substance; craving results when the individual is in situations reminiscent of heavy consumption

2. Consumption provides the individual with short-term rewards, reinforcing the consumption pattern

3. The individual ultimately comes to see no escape from an intolerable situation other than by ingesting one or more substances

IV. Alcohol abuse

A. Conditions associated with alcohol abuse

1. Alcohol withdrawal syndrome

a. Develops within 48 hours of the last drink

b. Produces vivid auditory hallucinations that usually last from a few hours to a few days but may persist for weeks or months

Nursing management of alcohol withdrawal

Most clients undergoing alcohol withdrawal exhibit telltale signs and symptoms during each withdrawal stage. The following chart lists the major signs and symptoms of each stage, along with appropriate nursing management.

STAGE	SIGNS AND SYMPTOMS	NURSING MANAGEMENT
I (within 8 hours after the last drink)	Mild tremors, diaphoresis, nausea, nervousness, tachycardia, increased blood pressure	• Carefully monitor the client's behavior. • Seek a physician's order for medication to relieve withdrawal symptoms. • Remain with the client once withdrawal begins, and talk with the client about the symptoms being experienced. • Monitor the client's vital signs.
II (8 to 10 hours after the last drink)	Increased tremors, hyperactivity, insomnia, anorexia, disorientation, delusions, visual hallucinations	• Administer medications, as ordered, to relieve withdrawal symptoms. • Remain with the client. • Keep the client oriented to reality. • Keep the environment free of distractions and unnecessary noise. • Regularly monitor the client's vital signs.
III (12 to 48 hours after the last drink)	Same as those listed for Stages I and II, plus persistent hallucinations; generalized tonic-clonic seizures also may occur	• Remain with the client. • Monitor vital signs. • Institute seizure precautions. • Administer anticonvulsant medications, as ordered. • Offer fluids and light foods, as tolerated, during periods of lucidity. • Maintain a peaceful environment.
IV (within 3 to 5 days after the last drink)	Delirium tremens, sleeplessness, hallucinations, tachycardia	• Remain with the client. • Monitor vital signs. • Maintain a peaceful environment. • Offer fluids and light foods, as tolerated, during periods of lucidity.

2. Alcohol withdrawal delirium (formerly called delirium tremens, or DTs)
   a. Develops within 72 hours of the last drink
   b. Occurs primarily in those who have been heavy drinkers for at least 5 years
   c. Produces visual hallucinations, paranoia, and disorientation (see *Nursing management of alcohol withdrawal*)

    3. Wernicke-Korsakoff syndrome
       a. Results from a deficiency in vitamin B complex
       b. Severely impairs cognitive functioning
       c. Produces peripheral neuropathy, cerebellar ataxia, confabulation, and myopathies

B. Physiologic effects of alcohol abuse
    1. Cardiovascular
       a. Cardiomyopathy
       b. Hypertension (increased systolic pressure)
    2. Gastrointestinal
       a. Cancer of oral mucosa
       b. Cirrhosis of the liver
       c. Colitis
       d. Decreased ability to absorb vitamins B_1 and B_{12}, resulting in malnutrition
       e. Esophageal varices
       f. Gastritis
       g. Pancreatitis
       h. Ulcers
    3. Genitourinary
       a. Impotence in males
       b. Loss of potassium from increased urine output
       c. Menstrual cycle disturbances in females
    4. Hematologic
       a. Anemia
       b. Hematomas
       c. Leukopenia
    5. Musculoskeletal
       a. Fractures
       b. Myopathies
    6. Neurologic
       a. Cerebral atrophy
       b. Impaired cognition and memory; blackouts
       c. Peripheral neuropathies
       d. Wernicke-Korsakoff syndrome
    7. Respiratory
       a. Chronic obstructive pulmonary disease
       b. Susceptibility to chronic infections

C. Screening tests to identify alcohol abuse
    1. CAGE questionnaire
       a. Consists of four questions
          (1) Have you ever felt you should cut down on your drinking?

(2) Have people annoyed you by criticizing your drinking?

(3) Have you ever felt bad or guilty about your drinking?

(4) Have you ever had a drink first thing in the morning to steady nerves or get rid of a hangover (eye-opener)?

 b. Indicates addiction with at least two affirmative responses

 2. Michigan Alcoholism Screening Test

  a. Consists of 26 items; points are allotted for affirmative responses

  b. Presumes alcoholism with four or more points (see page 88)

D. Continuum of alcohol consumption

 1. Experimental use: the first few times alcohol is ingested, the user is trying it out

 2. Responsible use: consumption is occasional and does no harm to the user

 3. Occasional misuse: consumption puts the user over the legal limit for intoxication on some occasions

 4. Early addiction (regular misuse): the person drinks to cope; intake is rapid; the person becomes preoccupied with alcohol, sneaks drinks, experiences hangovers, blackouts, and personality changes

 5. Middle addiction (middle dependency): the person sets out to drink; begins to lie about, feel guilty about, and make excuses for drinking; has blackouts more frequently; loses friends and interests; loses control over drinking

 6. Late addiction (late dependency): the person cannot do without alcohol; drinks until alcohol is gone, then searches for more; drinks to feel normal; alcohol becomes more important than anything in life; thinking becomes impaired; the person begins morning consumption

V. Drug abuse

A. Opiate (narcotic) abuse

 1. Morphine, meperidine, heroin, and codeine are the most commonly abused opiates

 2. Narcotic abusers quickly develop a tolerance for the narcotic, which increases the amount required to obtain the desired effect

 3. Physiologically, the individual experiences a reduced ability to feel pain, along with respiratory depression, drowsiness, and a diminution in gastrointestinal function

 4. Psychologically, the individual experiences a sense of extreme euphoria (or "high"), apathy, and impaired judgment

 5. A narcotics overdose causes respiratory and cardiovascular depression that can lead to coma and death

B. Cocaine abuse

 1. Effects are short-acting, lasting around 5 minutes when smoked as crack, 30 minutes when injected, and up to 90 minutes when inhaled

Michigan Alcoholism Screening Test (MAST)

Many health professionals rely on the Michigan Alcoholism Screening Test to determine the nature and severity of a client's alcohol abuse. To use this assessment tool, ask the client the questions in the left column. For each affirmative response (except where indicated by an asterisk), assign the number of points indicated in the right column; then total the points. Generally, a score of five or more points indicates alcoholism; a four-point total suggests alcoholism; and a score of three or less indicates that the client is not an alcoholic.

QUESTIONS	POINTS
1. Do you feel you are a normal drinker? (that is, do you drink less than or as much as most other people?)*	2
2. Have you ever awakened the morning after drinking the night before and found that you could not remember a part of the evening?	2
3. Does your spouse (or parents) ever worry or complain about your drinking?	1
4. Can you stop drinking without a struggle after one or two drinks?*	2
5. Do you ever feel guilty about your drinking?	1
6. Do friends and relatives think you are a normal drinker?*	2
7. Are you able to stop drinking when you want to?*	2
8. Have you ever attended a meeting of Alcoholics Anonymous (AA)?	5
9. Have you ever gotten into fights when drinking?	1
10. Has drinking ever created problems between you and your spouse (or parents)?	2
11. Has your spouse (or another family member) ever gone to anyone for help about your drinking?	2
12. Have you ever lost friends because of drinking?	2
13. Have you ever gotten into trouble at work or school because of drinking?	2
14. Have you ever lost a job because of drinking?	2
15. Have you ever neglected your obligations, your family, or your work for 2 or more days because you were drinking?	2
16. Do you drink before noon fairly often?	1
17. Have you ever been told that you have liver trouble? Cirrhosis?	2
18. After heavy drinking, have you ever had delirium tremens (DTs) or severe shaking, heard voices, or seen things that were not really there?	2
19. Have you ever gone to anyone for help about your drinking?	5

Michigan Alcoholism Screening Test (MAST) *(continued)*

QUESTIONS	POINTS
20. Have you ever been a patient in a psychiatric hospital or on a psychiatric ward of a general hospital when drinking was part of the problem that resulted in hospitalization?	5
21. Have you ever been seen at a psychiatric or mental health clinic or gone to any doctor, social worker, or counselor for help with an emotional problem that involved drinking?	2
22. Have you ever been arrested for driving while intoxicated?	2
23. Have you ever been arrested, even for a few hours, because of drunken behavior?	2

Source: Selzer, M.L. "The Michigan Alcoholism Screening Test: The Quest for a New Diagnostic Instrument," *American Journal of Psychiatry* 127(12): 1653-58, 1971. Used with permission.

  2. Physiologically, the individual experiences tachycardia, fever, and increased blood pressure and cardiac output
  3. Physiologic responses to cocaine can be severe; death has been associated with cocaine use
  4. Psychologically, the drug produces a sense of high energy, extreme euphoria, and marked increase in self-confidence; these effects make the drug extremely addictive

C. Benzodiazepine abuse
  1. Initially believed to be safe, these drugs were overprescribed for many years, causing many people to become dependent
  2. Psychologically, the drug produces euphoria, relaxation, and a sense of well-being
  3. Physiologically, the drug produces drowsiness, unsteady gait, and impaired verbal communication
  4. Withdrawal is potentially hazardous, sometimes resulting in seizures

D. Barbiturate abuse
  1. Long used as sedatives, barbiturates cause a reaction similar to that of alcohol
  2. Psychologically, the drugs create euphoria, depression, and, in some cases, hostile behavior
  3. Physiologically, the drugs exert a depressing effect on all body systems, especially reducing coordination
  4. Barbiturates combined with alcohol have a synergistic effect, potentially resulting in profound physiologic collapse

VI. Effects of addiction on life

A. Erosion of spiritual values and moral standards

B. Physical impairment, ranging from hangover to severe physiologic malfunctioning from organ damage

C. Mental deterioration, ranging from impaired judgment to severe dementia

D. Emotional symptoms, ranging from embarrassment to guilt, regret, and frequent use of defense mechanisms to justify abuse

E. Mounting family tensions as the abuser's behavior becomes more unpredictable and the family accommodates the abuser's behaviors

F. Dwindling circle of social friendships, eventually to include only fellow abusers

G. Sexual promiscuity

H. Reduction in leisure activities, with increasing amounts of time spent seeking out and consuming the substance

I. Financial problems, with increasing amounts of money diverted to procuring the substance

J. Legal difficulties as behavior deteriorates (such as driving under the influence or stealing to maintain the habit)

K. Occupational problems, with poor quality of work and unreliability sometimes resulting in termination

VII. Resources for abusers and their families

A. Support for abusers

   1. Alcoholics Anonymous (AA)

      a. Self-help group based on a 12-step program designed to help the individual remain abstinent

      b. Groups may be open (anyone may attend) or closed (only alcoholics may attend)

   2. Cocaine Anonymous (CA)

   3. Narcotics Anonymous (NA)

   4. Pills Anonymous (PA)

B. Support for families

   1. Adult Children of Alcoholics (ACoA): group for adults who need to work through unresolved issues related to growing up in an alcoholic home

   2. Al-Anon: support group for family members and friends of alcoholics; the group teaches its members about the disease of alcoholism and how to let the addicted member become responsible for self

   3. Alateen: support group for children aged 10 to 17; in this group, children of alcoholics can share experiences and learn how to deal with their alcoholic parents

VIII. Interventions in addiction disorders

A. Therapeutic intervention

    1. This is a technique for confronting abusers with their maladaptive behavior

    2. The goal is to get the abuser into a treatment program

    3. A therapeutic intervention consists of two important meetings

        a. In the first session, individuals important to the abuser (spouse, children, boss, friends, physician) meet with an intervention counselor to plan the intervention; during this meeting, which the abuser does not attend, the group agrees on what to say and how to say it

        b. During the second session, with the abuser present, those assembled express their concern for the individual; share examples of the abuser's behavior, thus acting as a mirror to the individual; and explain the consequences of not seeking immediate treatment (for instance, "You can't come home" or "You will not have a job")

    4. A carefully planned therapeutic intervention negates the abuser's main weapons — denial and manipulation — because all significant others are assembled in the same room

B. Detoxification

    1. Physical withdrawal from a chemical substance requires medical supervision to prevent physiologic collapse

    2. The purpose of detoxification is to prevent physical and emotional complications while the body undergoes withdrawal from the substance

C. In-facility treatment

    1. The individual resides at a special facility for a specified time, commonly from 21 to 30 days

    2. Education about substance abuse and group and individual therapy are emphasized

    3. In-facility treatment typically follows detoxification

D. Day treatment

    1. The individual stays at a treatment center during the day for individual and group activities

    2. Areas of emphasis include abstinence and change of life-style to maintain recovery

    3. Day treatment provides a support system during early recovery

E. Halfway house

    1. A halfway house provides a support system for addicts during the first few months of recovery (early recovery)

    2. The emphasis is on assuming responsibility for one's well-being

    3. Maintenance of the house is the responsibility of the residents

    4. Most residents are expected to find employment and adjust to living drug-free in the community

F. Alcoholics Anonymous

    1. AA emphasizes accepting and practicing the 12 steps for successful recovery from alcohol addiction

    2. New recoverers are encouraged to seek a sponsor to whom they can turn for support at any time

    3. Meetings are held daily, and members are advised to attend as many meetings weekly as needed to maintain sobriety

    4. Membership and attendance at meetings are strictly voluntary

    5. Because recovery is considered a lifelong process, many members attend meetings throughout their lives

G. Group therapy

    1. Group therapy enables the recovering addict to get feedback from peers

    2. It provides the addict with a temporary support system

H. Family therapy

    1. Because the addiction of one member disrupts the entire family and can lead to dysfunction, the primary emphasis is on helping the family unit to remain intact if family members desire it

    2. Members learn how to take care of themselves by setting realistic boundaries for behavior and by respecting the personal belongings of other members

    3. A specially trained family therapist assists members by discussing such issues as co-dependency and by encouraging re-enactments of family roles

I. Marital therapy

    1. In marital therapy, the spouses identify the ways in which addiction has affected their marriage

    2. They explore options for remaining together or separating

    3. The therapist aids the couple in their attempts to develop viable solutions to their problems

J. Behavior therapy

    1. In aversion therapy, the abuser experiences a negative sanction, such as vomiting, if consumption begins

        a. Disulfiram (Antabuse) is commonly prescribed for alcoholics during early recovery

        b. Because alcohol interacts with the drug to produce violent vomiting, the individual should not drink alcohol or use alcohol-containing products (such as aftershave) while taking disulfiram

    2. When stressed or tense, the individual can use relaxation techniques, which dissipate the automatic urge to consume the substance

Nursing management of substance abuse and withdrawal

When caring for a client who is suffering the effects of substance abuse, the nurse should be alert for signs of intoxication or withdrawal. As shown below, these signs can vary, depending on the substance ingested and the time of ingestion.

SUBSTANCE	SIGNS OF INTOXICATION	SIGNS OF WITHDRAWAL	NURSING IMPLICATIONS
Alcohol (beer, wine, liquor)	Labile affect, ataxia, impaired cognition, euphoria, diplopia, dysmetria, depressed mood, flushing, dry mouth, nystagmus, slurred speech, drowsiness, sense of floating, anorexia, violence	*Stage I:* Mild tremors, diaphoresis, nausea, nervousness, increased pulse rate and blood pressure	• Monitor the client's vital signs and behavior. • Seek a physician's order for a benzodiazepine to decrease withdrawal symptoms. • Remain with the client. • Promote sleep and rest.
		Stage II: Moderate to severe tremors, hyperactivity, insomnia, loss of appetite, disorientation, delusions, visual hallucinations	• Administer a benzodiazepine, as ordered. • Keep the environment quiet. • Remain with the client. • Monitor vital signs. • Orient the client to reality.
		Stage III: Persistent hallucinations, generalized tonic-clonic seizures	• Monitor vital signs. • Remain with the client. • Administer anticonvulsant medication, as ordered. • Offer fluids and light foods during periods of lucidity. • Keep the environment quiet and nonstimulating. • Institute seizure precautions.
		Stage IV: Alcohol withdrawal delirium, insomnia, hallucinations, tachycardia	• Remain with the client. • Monitor vital signs. • Keep the environment quiet. • Offer food and fluids during periods of lucidity.
Opiates (morphine, heroin)	Anxiety, impaired cognition, delirium, euphoria, flushing, sense of floating, hypotonia, pinhole pupils, skin picking, sleepiness, anorexia	Tearing (lacrimation), runny nose (rhinorrhea), excessive sweating, yawning, tachycardia, fever, insomnia, muscle aches, craving, nausea or vomiting, dilated pupils, chills	• Monitor vital signs. • Remain with the client. • Offer fluids and light foods as tolerated. • Keep the environment nondistracting and soothing. • Administer small doses of methadone, if ordered, to wean the client. *(continued)*

Nursing management of substance abuse and withdrawal (continued)

SUBSTANCE	SIGNS OF INTOXICATION	SIGNS OF WITHDRAWAL	NURSING IMPLICATIONS
CNS stimulants (amphetamines, cocaine, crack)	Labile affect, anxiety, anorexia, arrhythmia, restlessness, tremors, coryza, delirium, dizziness, euphoria, skin picking, violence, hallucinations, irritability, generalized tonic-clonic seizures, dry mouth, sleep disturbance, paresthesia, dilated pupils, hyperactive reflexes, tachycardia	Depression, fatigue, agitation, suicidal thoughts, paranoia, insomnia or hypersomnia, and (with amphetamines) disorientation	• Promote sleep and rest. • Monitor vital signs. • Monitor for suicidal ideation. • Administer an antidepressant, if ordered. • Remain with a frightened or disoriented client. • Orient the client to reality.
Hallucinogens (lysergic acid diethylamide [LSD], phencyclidine [PCP])	*LSD or PCP:* Hyperactive reflexes, restlessness, suspiciousness, tachycardia, hallucinations, labile affect, anorexia, body image changes, hypertension, dizziness, euphoria, sense of floating *LSD only:* Anxiety, sleep disturbance, tremors, dilated pupils *PCP only:* Slurred speech, blank stare, irritability, generalized tonic-clonic seizures, nystagmus, violence, vomiting, ataxia, delirium, depressed mood, dysmetria	*LSD:* None *PCP:* Depression, lethargy, craving	• Institute safety precautions.
Cannabis (marijuana)	Slowed speech, apathy, slowed reflexes, reduced inhibitions, altered state of awareness, red eyes, dry mouth, memory loss, lethargy	Anxiety, restlessness	• Help a client with memory loss to fill in gaps of information. • Attend to self-care needs that a lethargic or apathetic client may have neglected.
Barbiturates and anxiolytics (diazepam, pentobarbital)	Drowsiness, euphoria, fatigue, sense of floating, hypotonia, orthostatic hypotension, irritability, anorexia, anxiety, slurred speech, ataxia, poor memory and comprehension, seizures, delirium, depressed mood, diplopia, dizziness, dysmetria, nystagmus, violence	Nausea or vomiting; generalized malaise; tachycardia; excessive sweating; anxiety; irritability; orthostatic hypotension; coarse tremors of hands, tongue, and eyelids; insomnia; generalized tonic-clonic seizures	• Monitor vital signs. • Remain with the client. • Promote sleep and rest. • Offer fluids and light foods as tolerated. • Administer medications, if ordered, to wean the client. • Institute seizure precautions.

3. Relapse prevention involves teaching the individual to recognize and avoid the cues that lead to consumption; in some instances, old friends must be avoided and new friendships cultivated

4. Assertiveness training shows the individual how to feel empowered without relying on a substance

K. Employee assistance programs

1. Business firms have set up special programs that provide professional care to employees who suffer from substance dependence

2. Education and ongoing support from co-workers and the employer are available to the employee during recovery; responsibility in the workplace is emphasized

IX. **Levels of addiction prevention**

A. *Primary prevention* focuses on preventing substance abuse, usually through education programs aimed at children and adolescents

B. *Secondary prevention* focuses on early identification of and intervention with substance abusers to prevent recurrence

C. *Tertiary prevention* focuses on rehabilitation to prevent recurrence (for additional information, see *Nursing management of substance abuse and withdrawal,* page 93)

Clinical situation

Jim Curry, age 41, is brought to the emergency department (ED) by his girlfriend, who says Jim vomited what looked like coffee grounds about 20 minutes earlier. The ED physician decides to admit him to the hospital for diagnostic testing. When Jim arrives on your nursing unit, you notice that he looks older than his stated age. He's pale and diaphoretic. He is 5'10" tall and weighs 150 lb. Your assessment reveals the following: temperature, 100° F; pulse rate, 120 beats/minute; blood pressure, 146/100 mm Hg; clear lung sounds; slightly distended abdomen; slightly yellow sclera.

As part of your nursing assessment, you ask Jim about his use of substances. He states that he smokes two packs of cigarettes per day, drinks four to five cups of coffee in the morning only, and consumes "a little beer" every day. When you ask Jim to quantify "a little beer," he says, "Maybe a can or two." He begins to squirm when you ask whether he uses other substances. "I don't do any hard stuff. I might smoke pot once in a while — just to mellow out. Pot isn't harmful, you know. Most people just don't understand how it works."

Because Jim says he feels nauseated, you decide to let him rest. You tell him you will be leaving soon and that another nurse will be caring for him during the evening. At 10 p.m., Jim asks the evening nurse for "something for my nerves." Jim is mildly tremulous and perspiring. His pulse rate is 130 beats/minute, and his blood pressure is 158/120 mm Hg. Suspecting that Jim might be experiencing early stage alcohol withdrawal, the nurse confers with the supervisor, who arranges to transfer Jim immediately to the hospital's detoxification unit.

Assessment (nursing behaviors and rationales)

1. Assess changes in Jim's physiologic status. *Increased pulse rate and blood pressure signal Stage I of alcohol withdrawal syndrome.*

2. Assess Jim's level of orientation. *Fluctuating levels of orientation signal Stage II withdrawal. Preventing late-stage alcohol withdrawal syndrome will be a top priority.*

3. Assess Jim for anxiety and alcohol hallucinosis. *Physical signs resulting from withdrawal can produce moderate to severe anxiety levels. Withdrawal causes the client to misperceive external stimuli, resulting in misinterpretation of what is really happening (hallucinosis).*

4. Assess Jim's nutritional status. *Drinking bouts may have caused the client to develop poor eating habits, causing vitamin deficiencies and electrolyte imbalances.*

Nursing diagnoses
• High risk for injury related to confusion and unsteadiness
• Altered nutrition (less than body requirements) related to poor eating habits
• Sleep pattern disturbance related to alcohol withdrawal
• Disorientation and confusion related to misperceptions of external stimuli

Planning and goals
• Jim will not injure himself while on the detoxification unit.
• Jim will not experience Stage II withdrawal.
• Jim will reestablish a nutritious diet.
• Jim will be less confused and will have fewer misperceptions of external stimuli.

Implementation (nursing behaviors and rationales)

1. Provide one-on-one monitoring as long as Jim's condition is unstable. *One-on-one monitoring ensures the continuous assessment necessary for calibration of medication to control withdrawal and to provide a safe environment.*

2. Administer medication (usually a benzodiazepine), as prescribed. *Jim's physician has prescribed lorazepam (Ativan) 2 mg every 8 hours on the first day, 1 mg every 8 hours on the second day, and 0.5 mg every 8 hours on the third day, along with thiamine 100 mg I.M. for 3 days. Lorazepam is administered to prevent acute alcohol withdrawal syndrome. Because this client may have liver damage, lorazepam is the benzodiazepine of choice because of its short half-life. Thiamine promotes the body's ability to utilize carbohydrates fully.*

3. Document Jim's response to lorazepam. *If the ordered dosage is not effective, the physician will need to increase it. Preventing second-stage withdrawal is necessary for the client's safety.*

4. Maintain a quiet, peaceful environment by speaking softly, dimming the lights in Jim's room, and screening out noises. *A quiet, peaceful environment promotes rest and enhances the medication's sedative qualities.*

5. While acknowledging his feelings and experiences, reassure Jim that visual hallucinations (such as animals or insects) are not real. Provide emotional support. *Emphasizing reality, acknowledging the client's feelings, and providing em-*

pathy are crucial to helping the client through the first phase of alcohol with-drawal syndrome.

Evaluation
• Jim completes detoxification without incident.
• Jim does not experience second-stage withdrawal.

Clinical situation
(continued)

Before Jim leaves the detoxification unit, his physician, girlfriend, and two children participate in a therapeutic intervention with him. As a result of the intervention, Jim reluctantly agrees to transfer to an inpatient treatment setting.

Medical records sent from the hospital to the inpatient treatment setting reveal that Jim's hemoglobin level was 10 g/dl. Toxicology screening showed that when Jim entered the hospital, his blood alcohol level was 0.23 and his urine was positive for cannabis. Jim's gamma-glutamyl transpeptidase (GGTP) test reveals liver damage.

On his first day in the treatment setting, Jim completes the CAGE questionnaire, answering the second and fourth questions affirmatively. However, Jim is adamant that his alcohol consumption is not unreasonable. "After all, I only drink beer."

During the next 2 weeks, Jim attends multiple individual and group sessions, as well as classes in which the disease of alcoholism is explained. Jim reluctantly participates in these activities. He manages self-care but has lost 3 lb because he "just isn't hungry." Jim's counselor learns that Jim consumes up to 12 cans of beer daily and uses cannabis three times weekly. Jim states that he has always been able to drink more than most people. When asked about hangovers, Jim replies that he used to get them but hasn't had any bad hangovers for at least 5 years. When asked about family history, Jim reveals that his father, uncles, and grandfather were "heavy drinkers." He says his mother never consumed alcohol.

Assessment *(nursing behaviors and rationales)*

1. Monitor Jim's physical condition, especially noting hemoglobin level, weight and appetite, and signs of jaundice. *Medical evidence proves that the client's prolonged use of alcohol has damaged his body. Physical problems must be corrected to ensure the client's physical well-being and to prevent further damage. Lower-level needs must be met first.*

2. Assess Jim's use of denial. *The nurse must determine Jim's progress toward understanding that he has an alcohol problem and that he must take responsibility for his recovery.*

Nursing diagnoses
• Ineffective denial related to the client's consumption pattern
• Altered nutrition (less than body requirements) related to lack of appetite, gastric ulcer, and deteriorating physical health

Planning and goals
• Jim will state at least three effects that alcohol has had on his body.

- Jim will consume nutritional foods offered and will attain a weight of at least 150 lb.

Implementation (nursing behaviors and rationales)

1. Explain the alcohol-use continuum, and ask Jim to place himself along that continuum (see section IV-D on page 87). *This activity will encourage the client to look objectively at how alcohol has affected his life.*

2. Review the CAGE questionnaire with Jim. *Discussing how others view his alcohol consumption and how he needs alcohol early in the day chips away at the wall of denial he has erected.*

3. Have Jim attend meetings with alcohol-abuse peers who have moved beyond denial. *What peers say commonly carries more weight than what health care professionals say.*

4. Provide Jim with a menu of nutritious foods, and ask him to indicate his preferences. *An appropriate diet will help correct nutritional deficiencies. The client will be more likely to follow the diet if it contains foods that he enjoys.*

5. Offer small quantities of nutritious food every 3 hours. *A client who does not feel well usually cannot eat a lot at one time. Keeping food in the stomach will absorb gastric acids. The client's ability to maintain a healthy weight depends on the amount of food he ingests.*

Evaluation

- Jim recognizes the effects that alcohol has had on his body.
- Jim weighs 151 lb and consumes the food offered to him.

Clinical situation
(continued)

Jim Curry has been in treatment for 16 days. Today, during a rather intense group session, Jim tells the group about his two failed marriages, his strained relationships with his 14- and 17-year-old children, and numerous jobs lost over the past 20 years. He further relays how he contracted genital herpes 5 years ago during a blackout. With great feeling, Jim says he regrets the years he has wasted, the hardships he has imposed on others, and his flagrant disregard of the values he once held dear. He shakes his head sadly and says, "I don't know if I can ever be forgiven for all the damage I've done."

Assessment (nursing behaviors and rationales)

1. Assess Jim's coping skills. *Jim has used alcohol and marijuana in the past to cope with stress. If he has no legitimate coping skills, he will need to learn new ones to prevent relapse or suicide.*

2. Assess Jim's support system, including spiritual values. *Without an adequate support system, the potential for relapse increases.*

3. Assess what Jim wants to accomplish sober that he could not accomplish while abusing alcohol and marijuana. *This provides Jim with structure during recovery and allows the nurse to evaluate how well Jim can set attainable goals.*

4. Assess Jim's sexual practices and his knowledge about sexually transmitted diseases (STDs). *A client with genital herpes must have accurate information to control the contagious disease. The client also is at risk for contracting other STDs.*

Nursing diagnoses

- Altered role performance related to impaired judgment and developmental immaturity
- Spiritual distress related to engaging in behaviors contrary to the client's core value system
- Altered sexuality pattern related to contracting an STD

Planning and goals

- Jim will identify behaviors appropriate for parenting, intimate sexual relationships, employment, and social relationships.
- Jim will identify the core values most important to him.
- Jim will describe how to protect others from contracting genital herpes and how to protect himself against other STDs.

Implementation (nursing behaviors and rationales)

1. Enroll Jim in parenting classes. *These classes will enable the client to develop effective parenting skills, thereby enhancing his ability to relate with his children in a mutually rewarding way.*

2. Have Jim attend an ACoA meeting. *In this group, the client will learn how his father's alcoholism affected him as a child and as an adult. Additionally, he will have opportunities to build a support system and to relate to others with similar experiences.*

3. Role-play various life situations with Jim, focusing on situations that would create stress in everyday life. *The client's past coping skills have proven to be limited and ineffective; role-playing is a safe way for the client to develop the new skills he'll need to remain sober.*

4. Have Jim attend AA at least three times a week during the first few months of recovery. *Adequate support can help prevent relapse, which is more likely to occur during the first year of recovery than at any other time. AA is a spiritually based self-help group that will assist the client in reestablishing spiritual balance in his life and provide him with emotional support. He will learn how to make peace with himself and those important to him.*

5. Teach Jim the importance of practicing safe sex, including condom use and avoidance of anal sex and body fluid intake. Explain that abstinence from sex is the only certain way to prevent the spread of STDs and that maintaining a monogamous relationship is safer than engaging in sex with multiple partners. *Knowledge of safe sexual practices contributes to the well-being of the client and sexual partners.*

6. Teach Jim how to manage genital herpes if he doesn't already know how. *This is important to the client's physical and social well-being.*

7. Have Jim role-play how to tell his sex partners that he has genital herpes. *The client will be more likely to inform future partners if he has practiced how to do this and is comfortable with it.*

Evaluation

- Jim enrolls in a class for parents of teenagers.
- Jim has found a job in his area of expertise.

- Jim has developed friendships with others in his ACoA and AA groups and plans to join them on social occasions.
- Jim is learning how to accept and practice the 12 steps of the recovery program. He says he feels good about the progress he is beginning to make.
- Jim has attended classes on human sexuality and can describe safe sexual practices. Jim has discussed his herpes with his girlfriend. They practice safe sex, and she remains free of the disease.
- Jim and his girlfriend have elected to attend two to four sessions with a counselor to sort out their relationship.

11 Adjustment disorder

I. Overview

    A. Adjustment disorder is characterized by a maladaptive reaction to a psychosocial stressor that can be readily identified

        1. The reaction is considered maladaptive under certain circumstances

            a. Social or occupational (including school) functioning is markedly impaired

            b. The symptoms exhibited are exaggerated beyond the usual expected response to the severity of the stressor

            c. The response does not meet the criteria for any other mental disorder and is neither an isolated incident nor uncomplicated bereavement (see *Diagnostic criteria for adjustment disorder,* page 102)

        2. The maladaptive reaction occurs within 3 months after the onset of the stressor and cannot have lasted longer than 6 months

    B. Clinicians recognize nine types of adjustment disorder, classified by the predominant symptom or group of symptoms displayed (see *Types of adjustment disorder,* page 104)

        1. Although many of the types described are similar to other psychiatric diagnoses, they are only partial syndromes of other mental disorders

        2. For example, adjustment disorder with depressed mood and adjustment disorder with anxious mood are not severe enough to be diagnosed as anxiety or depression

    C. Behavioral reactions to stress are expected to remit soon after the stressor ceases or, in cases of continued stress, when a new level of adaptation is reached

II. Theoretical perspectives

    A. Biological theory

        1. Problems result from biochemical imbalances in the brain

        2. The midbrain releases norepinephrine, which causes severe anxiety (see Chapter 3)

Diagnostic criteria for adjustment disorder

The following chart presents the *DSM-III-R* diagnostic criteria for adjustment disorder.

A. The disturbance must represent a maladaptive reaction to an identifiable psychosocial stressor and must occur within 3 months of the stressor's onset

B. The maladaptive nature of the reaction is indicated by either of the following:
   1. Impaired functioning on the job, at school, in usual social activities, or in relationships with others
   2. Symptoms that exceed normal and expected reactions to the stressor

C. The disturbance is not part of a pattern of overreaction to stress nor an exacerbation of another mental disorder

D. The disturbance has persisted for no longer than 6 months

E. The disturbance does not meet the criteria for any specific mental disorder and does not represent uncomplicated bereavement

Source: *Diagnostic and Statistical Manual of Mental Disorders,* Third Edition-Revised. Washington, D.C.: American Psychiatric Association, 1987. Adapted with permission.

   B. Psychodynamic theory
   1. Hidden psychological conflicts cause anxiety
   2. This stimulates a maladaptive response to stress in an individual who:
      a. Cannot complete appropriate developmental tasks
      b. Has unmet dependency needs
      c. Is fixated in an earlier developmental level
      d. Has retarded ego development

   C. Interpersonal theory
   1. Problems result when an individual's expectations or needs are not met in interpersonal relationships with significant others
   2. Unsatisfactory early interpersonal relationships (for instance, early separation from one's mother) can lead to problems with adjustment in later life

   D. Behavioral theory
   1. Maladaptive behavior is learned
   2. Negative learning patterns experienced by the individual have impeded the development of self-esteem and effective coping skills

III. General nursing assessments

   A. Assess the time, duration, and nature of the stressor
   1. The client usually reports a psychosocial stressor occurring in the 3 months before the onset of symptoms
   2. If symptoms last longer than 6 months, another mental disorder should be considered

3. The symptoms may stem from a single stressor (such as loss of a job) or from multiple stressors (such as business difficulties and marital problems)

4. Although some stressors are easily identified (divorce or the death of a loved one), others are less evident (going away to school, leaving the parental home, and other developmental milestones)

5. The stressor may be recurrent (such as a seasonal business crisis) or continuous (such as poverty, chronic illness, a natural disaster, strained family relationships, and religious or racial prejudice)

B. Assess any impairment in social or occupational functioning for symptoms beyond the normal and expected reactions to the stressor

1. The client appears tearful and jittery

2. The client expresses anger inappropriately through fighting, vandalism, or reckless driving

3. School or work performance declines

4. Use or abuse of psychoactive substances increases

5. Complaints of headache, backache, and fatigue arise

C. Assess for feelings of inadequacy, low self-esteem, and difficulty adapting to change

D. Assess the client's pre-illness ability to cope with day-to-day problems

IV. Possible nursing diagnoses

A. Anxiety related to loss of control over life

B. Impaired adjustment related to recent change in life

C. Ineffective individual coping related to low self-esteem

D. Self-esteem disturbance related to feelings of inadequacy

E. Altered role performance related to inability to solve problems

F. Powerlessness related to inability to cope

V. Psychotherapeutic goals and treatments

A. Most individuals with an adjustment disorder are treated on an outpatient basis; treatment depends on the symptoms exhibited

B. Priorities include providing for safety needs, lessening anxiety, and identifying problem-solving and coping mechanisms

C. Treatment should not last longer than is necessary to relieve symptoms

D. Treatment goals include restoring the client's level of functioning to a pre-illness level and promoting behavioral changes to strengthen that part of the client's personality still vulnerable to stress

Types of adjustment disorder

The following chart presents the nine types of adjustment disorder, as classified by *DSM-III-R.*

Adjustment Disorder with Anxious Mood

Predominant manifestations include such symptoms as nervousness, worry, and jitteriness.

Adjustment Disorder with Depressed Mood

Predominant manifestations include such symptoms as depressed mood, tearfulness, and feelings of hopelessness.

Adjustment Disorder with Disturbance of Conduct

Predominant manifestation is conduct that violates either the rights of others or major age-appropriate societal norms and rules (for example, truancy, vandalism, reckless driving, fighting, or defaulting on legal responsibilities).

Adjustment Disorder with Mixed Disturbance of Emotions and Conduct

Predominant manifestations include emotional symptoms (such as depression or anxiety) and disturbance of conduct (see above).

Adjustment Disorder with Mixed Emotional Features

Predominant manifestation is a combination of depression and anxiety or other emotions (such as an adolescent who, after moving away from home and parental supervision, reacts with ambivalence, depression, anger, and signs of increased dependence). The major differential is with depressive and anxiety disorders.

Adjustment Disorder with Physical Complaints

Predominant manifestations include physical symptoms (such as fatigue, headache, backache, or other aches and pains) that are not diagnosable as a specific Axis III disorder or condition.

Adjustment Disorder with Withdrawal

Predominant manifestation is social withdrawal without significantly depressed or anxious mood.

Adjustment Disorder with Work (or Academic) Inhibition

Predominant manifestation is an inhibition in work or academic functioning (such as an inability to study or to write papers or reports) occurring in a person whose previous work or academic performance has been adequate. Anxiety and depression also are common.

Adjustment Disorder Not Otherwise Specified

Disorders involving maladaptive reactions to psychosocial stressors that are not classifiable as specific types of adjustment disorder.

Source: *Diagnostic and Statistical Manual of Mental Disorders,* Third Edition-Revised. Washington, D.C.: American Psychiatric Association, 1987. Adapted with permission.

E. Individual psychotherapy is the most common treatment for adjustment disorders

    1. Its goal is to replace the client's maladaptive response with a more effective one

    2. Three widely used types of psychotherapy are psychodynamic therapy, behavioral therapy, and family therapy

        a. Psychodynamic therapy

            (1) The client's problem results from negative self-image, early psychological trauma, or inadequate personality development

            (2) The therapist uses supportive and expressive psychodynamic techniques to help the client resolve the problem

        b. Behavioral therapy

            (1) The client's problem results from patterns of maladaptive responses to situations

            (2) Coaching, modeling, and reinforcement schedules are some of the psychotherapeutic techniques used to help the client correct ineffective responses to stress

        c. Family therapy

            (1) This type of therapy directs treatment away from the client and toward the client's family unit

            (2) Its goal is to change the social network function

VI. General nursing interventions

    A. Monitor for suicide potential

        1. Ask the client direct questions about any intent, plan, and means to do self-harm

        2. Provide a safe environment, placing potentially harmful objects out of reach

    B. Help the client identify thoughts and feelings associated with the change in life or current situational crisis

        1. Encourage the client to express feelings, including sadness and anger

        2. Explore how to handle frustration or pent-up anger in socially acceptable ways (walking briskly, engaging in a sporting event, hitting a punching bag)

    C. Teach the client relaxation techniques, and have the client practice them under your supervision

    D. Determine which stage of grief (and associated behaviors) the client may be experiencing; teach the client about these stages and behaviors (see Chapter 3)

    E. Help the client determine aspects of personal life still under the client's control

        1. Encourage the client to perform self-care, to set goals, and to make independent decisions

2. Help the client identify methods of coping or problem solving that proved successful in the past

3. Assist the client in using the problem-solving process to explore alternatives and to select more adaptive strategies of coping with stress

F. Refer the client to an appropriate support group, such as Alcoholics Anonymous or a bereavement group

Clinical situation

Pamela Jones, age 32, is a well-groomed legal secretary who comes to the outpatient clinic where you are on duty. She tells you that she has come on the advice of a co-worker. She has been experiencing frequent bouts of crying and states that she feels like she is "unlikable." She has canceled all her usual social engagements and is no longer attending her aerobics class, which she previously enjoyed. Pamela states that her symptoms began about 1 month ago, after she discovered that Tom, a man she had been dating (and had expected to marry), was married and no longer wanted to see her.

Assessment (nursing behaviors and rationales)

1. Conduct a health history and physical examination. Question Pamela about alcohol and drug use, and pay special attention to current eating habits. *Any deterioration in physical health will need attention, and physical causes for symptoms must be ruled out. Severe depression can lead to changes in eating and sleeping patterns; clients typically use psychoactive substances as a coping mechanism in stressful situations.*

2. Conduct a psychosocial assessment to assess suicide potential, available social supports, occupational and financial stressors, and previous losses. Determine which coping skills the client uses when under stress. *A psychosocial assessment will assist in determining the severity of the client's reaction to the situation, along with client strengths that may be useful in establishing a treatment plan.*

3. Determine the client's perception of the situation. *The nurse must understand how the client perceives the problem in order to establish a client-specific treatment plan.*

Nursing diagnoses

• Dysfunctional grieving related to a real or perceived loss
• Ineffective individual coping related to a situational crisis
• Impaired social interaction related to negative self-image

Planning and goals

• Pamela Jones will express her thoughts and feelings about this loss to her close friends.
• She will identify alternate coping skills to handle stress.

Implementation (nursing behaviors and rationales)

1. Actively involve Pamela in the physical and psychosocial assessment. *This not only provides the data necessary to plan care but also lets Pamela know that, as an active participant in her treatment, she has some control over the situation.*

2. Help Pamela identify her thoughts and feelings about the dissolution of her relationship with Tom, including negative and positive aspects of the change. *The client may need help in viewing the change objectively because the change can have both positive and negative consequences. Her perception of the event is particularly important and needs to be explored in relation to the actual event.*

3. Encourage her to express openly any anger or sadness. *This allows Pamela to acknowledge and begin to deal with her feelings. The nurse's acceptance of these expressions helps the client recognize that anger and sadness are normal rather than "bad."*

4. Explore alternative physical outlets that Pamela can rely on to diffuse anger and hostility. *Physical exercise provides a safe and effective way to release pent-up emotions.*

5. Explain the stages of grief to Pamela, including the behaviors commonly associated with each stage. *Grieving over the loss of a close relationship is normal and socially accepted. Knowing this may help relieve some of the anxiety and guilt that these responses commonly generate.*

6. Encourage Pamela to review her relationship with Tom. With sensitivity and support, help her to examine the reality of a romantic situation in which one partner makes misrepresentations. *The client must give up idealized perceptions and be able to accept both positive and negative aspects of the situation before she can complete the grieving process.*

7. Assist Pamela in identifying areas of strength and previous coping abilities. *Focusing on past success enhances the client's self-esteem and provides a blueprint for resolving the present crisis.*

8. Teach Pamela to solve problems one step at a time. *Clients benefit from learning the steps of a logical and orderly process to solving problems. Recognition of personal control, however minimal, diminishes the sense of powerlessness and promotes a positive self-image.*

9. Encourage Pamela to discuss the situation with a trusted friend. *Interacting with an important person in the client's life limits opportunities for isolation. Additionally, feedback from peers may help the client correct misperceptions of the event and learn new coping behaviors.*

Evaluation

- Pamela Jones remained in therapy for 10 weeks.
- She resumed social contacts with friends and returned to her aerobics class.
- Confiding in her best friend, Pamela was able to express her anger at Tom's deception and her sadness about the loss of a possible marriage partner.

12

Dissociative disorders

I. Overview

    A. Dissociative disorders are characterized by a sudden disruption in consciousness, memory, identity, or sense of reality

    B. Severe anxiety and psychic conflict are common precursors, and sometimes a dissociative disorder develops after a major trauma that has caused the victim to fear for his or her life

    C. Although dissociative disorders are uncommon, their occurrence produces dramatic disruptions of the individual's personality

II. Multiple personality disorder (MPD)

    A. Characteristics

        1. Two or more distinct personalities, or personality states, existing within the same person

            a. At least two of the personalities take full control of the person's behavior at various times

            b. The transition from one personality to another usually occurs within seconds to minutes

            c. The personalities usually are aware of some or all of the others in varying degrees

            d. The client may report memory gaps or lost periods of time during which another personality is in control

        2. Severe, often violent acting-out behaviors

        3. Self-mutilation and suicide attempts

        4. History of frequent admissions to a psychiatric facility

        5. History of physical or sexual abuse or severe emotional trauma sometime during childhood

    B. Criteria for medical diagnosis (see the *DSM-III-R* diagnostic criteria for multiple personality disorder on page 112)

    C. Treatment (aims to reintegrate the personalities into one person who can function effectively in society)

        1. Psychoanalytic psychotherapy (treatment of choice)

        2. Hypnosis (can be a helpful tool)

        3. Drug therapy (to relieve associated anxiety and depression)

        4. In-patient admission (may be necessary when the client's safety or the safety of others is at risk)

D. Possible nursing diagnoses

    1. Ineffective individual and family coping related to inability to deal with multiple personalities

    2. High risk for injury related to suicidal or homicidal impulses

    3. Post-trauma response related to childhood abuse or trauma

E. General nursing interventions

    1. Maintain a safe environment; take all necessary safety precautions to protect the client, other clients, and staff during periods of acting out

    2. Educate unit personnel about the course and treatment of this disorder

    3. Carefully evaluate any participation in the treatment plan by family members (severely dysfunctional families are typically involved in the etiology of this disorder)

    4. Administer medications as ordered, and evaluate their effectiveness

    5. Observe and document any personalities that emerge and any precursors to their emergence

III. Psychogenic fugue

A. Characteristics

    1. Sudden, unexpected (though apparently purposeful) travel away from home or work, followed by an inability to recall one's past

    2. Adoption by the client of a new identity (either partial or complete)

    3. Possible confusion or disorientation

    4. Heavy alcohol use (possible predisposing factor)

    5. Severe personal or environmental stress (such as a natural disaster or a war) preceding the psychogenic fugue

    6. Spontaneous, rapid recovery

B. Criteria for medical diagnosis (see the *DSM-III-R* diagnostic criteria for psychogenic fugue on page 112)

C. Possible nursing diagnoses

    1. Ineffective individual coping related to memory loss

    2. High risk for injury related to disorientation

    3. Personal identity disturbance related to loss of old identity and adoption of new one

D. Treatment

    1. Thorough investigation of underlying stressors

    2. Psychotherapy (if necessary)

E. General nursing interventions

    1. Maintain a safe environment during the fugue state

    2. Reorient the client to time, place, and person during recovery

    3. Involve the client's support systems in identifying predisposing stressors

      4. Arrange opportunities for the client to discuss precipitating factors and feelings about having experienced this disorder, using one-on-one nurse-client interactions, support groups, or ongoing psychotherapy

IV. Psychogenic amnesia

  A. Characteristics

      1. Sudden memory loss of important personal information

         a. The memory loss is more significant than simple forgetfulness

         b. The memory loss is not attributable to an organic mental disorder

      2. Onset usually after severe psychological stress (sometimes after the threat of physical injury or death)

      3. Purposeless wandering, disorientation, and confusion

      4. Abrupt and complete recovery (recurrences are rare)

      5. Remembrance of the memory loss after recovery

  B. Types

      1. Localized (or circumscribed) memory loss: inability to remember events that occurred during a circumscribed time, usually after a severely traumatic incident (the most common type)

      2. Selective memory loss: inability to remember some of the events that occurred during a circumscribed time

      3. Generalized amnesia: inability to remember anything about one's life

      4. Continuous amnesia: inability to recall any events that occurred after a specific time, up to and including the present

  C. Criteria for medical diagnosis (see the *DSM-III-R* diagnostic criteria for psychogenic amnesia on page 112)

  D. Treatment

      1. Supportive care during the amnesia episode

      2. Psychotherapy afterward, if indicated (to assist in identifying precipitating stressors and in building new coping skills)

  E. Possible nursing diagnoses

      1. Ineffective individual coping related to memory loss

      2. High risk for injury related to confusion and wandering

      3. Personal identity disturbance related to inability to recall the past

  F. General nursing interventions

      1. Maintain a safe environment during the amnesia episode

      2. Reorient the client to reality, as needed

      3. Offer opportunities for the client to discuss precipitating events

      4. Provide support for the client and significant others during recovery

V. Depersonalization disorder

A. Characteristics

    1. Persistent or recurrent and distressing alteration in perception of one's sense of self, such that one's sense of reality is temporarily lost or changed

    2. Feelings of detachment (as if an outside observer of oneself) or of being in a mechanical or dreamlike state

    3. Various types of sensory anesthesia, commonly accompanied by feelings of not being in control of one's actions

    4. Associated features

        a. Derealization

        b. Alteration in one's perception of surroundings

        c. Lost awareness of the external world

        d. Dizziness

        e. Depression

        f. Anxiety

        g. Somatic complaints

        h. Fear of going insane

        i. Disturbances in time and memory

    5. Rapid onset of symptoms

    6. Intact reality testing

    7. Single, brief episode commonly following severe stress (may occur in as many as 70% of adolescents and young adults)

B. Criteria for medical diagnosis (see the *DSM-III-R* diagnostic criteria for depersonalization disorder on page 112)

C. Treatment

    1. Psychotherapy and supportive measures on an outpatient basis

    2. Antidepressant or antianxiety medications

D. Possible nursing diagnoses

    1. Anxiety related to feelings of lost perception

    2. Ineffective individual coping related to fear of going insane

    3. Self-esteem disturbance related to inability to deal with events

    4. Sensory-perceptual alteration (visual, auditory, kinesthetic, gustatory, tactile, olfactory) related to sensory anesthesia

E. General nursing interventions

    1. Engage the client in a supportive, one-on-one relationship to alleviate anxiety and worry

    2. Help the client identify any stressors that may have precipitated the incident

    3. Assist the client in identifying and developing more effective ways of coping with stress

Diagnostic criteria for dissociative disorders

The following chart presents the *DSM-III-R* diagnostic criteria for the dissociative disorders discussed in this chapter.

Multiple personality disorder
A. Two or more distinct personalities or personality states (each with its own relatively enduring pattern of perceiving, relating to, and thinking about the environment and self) exist within the individual
B. At least two of these personalities or personality states recurrently take full control of the person's behavior

Psychogenic fugue
A. The predominant disturbance is sudden, unexpected travel away from home or one's customary place of work, with inability to recall one's past
B. The individual assumes a new identity (partial or complete)
C. The disturbance is not due to multiple personality disorder or to an organic mental disorder (for example, partial complex seizures in temporal lobe epilepsy)

Psychogenic amnesia
A. The predominant disturbance is an episode of sudden inability to recall important personal information that is too extensive to be explained by ordinary forgetfulness
B. The disturbance is not due to multiple personality disorder or to an organic mental disorder (for example, blackouts during alcohol intoxication)

Depersonalization disorder
A. The individual experiences persistent or recurrent episodes of depersonalization, as indicated by either of the following:
  1. Feeling detached from, and as if one is an outside observer of, one's mental processes or body
  2. Feeling like an automaton or as if in a dream
B. During the depersonalization experience, reality testing remains intact
C. The depersonalization is sufficiently severe and persistent to cause marked distress
D. The depersonalization experience is the predominant disturbance and is not a symptom of another disorder (such as schizophrenia, panic disorder, or agoraphobia without history of panic disorder but with limited symptom attacks of depersonalization) or temporal lobe epilepsy

Dissociative disorder not otherwise specified
Any disorder in which the predominant feature is a dissociative symptom (that is, a disturbance or alteration in the normally integrative functions of identity, memory, or consciousness) that does not meet the criteria for a specific dissociative disorder. Examples follow.
  1. Ganser syndrome: the giving of "approximate answers" to questions, commonly associated with other symptoms, such as amnesia, disorientation, perceptual disturbances, fugue, and conversion symptoms

Diagnostic criteria for dissociative disorders *(continued)*

2. Cases in which more than one personality state can assume executive control of the individual, but not more than one personality state is sufficiently distinct to meet the full criteria for multiple personality disorder, or cases in which a second personality never assumes complete executive control
3. Trance states (altered states of consciousness with markedly diminished or selectively focused responsiveness to environmental stimuli); in children, this may follow physical abuse or trauma
4. Derealization unaccompanied by depersonalization
5. Dissociated states that may occur in people who have been subjected to periods of prolonged and intense coercive persuasion (such as brainwashing, thought reform, or indoctrination while the captive of terrorists or cultists)
6. Cases in which sudden, unexpected travel and organized, purposeful behavior with inability to recall one's past are not accompanied by the assumption of a new identity, partial or complete

Source: *Diagnostic and Statistical Manual of Mental Disorders,* Third Edition-Revised. Washington, D.C.: American Psychiatric Association, 1987. Adapted with permission.

---

4. Teach the client when to administer medications prescribed for anxiety or depression
5. Assist the client in achieving effective reality testing and in maintaining a sense of self; encourage self-care and the expression of perceptions and feelings about the current situation

VI. Dissociative disorders not otherwise specified (NOS)

A. These disorders have a predominant dissociative symptom but do not meet the specific criteria of any one dissociative disorder (see the *DSM-III-R* diagnostic criteria in the chart above)

B. Treatment, possible nursing diagnoses, and general nursing interventions are similar to those for other dissociative disorders

Clinical situation

Sue, an 18-year-old college freshman, presents at the University Health Center asking for a mental health consultation. She reports, hesitantly but with great anxiety, that in the 3 months since college began, she has increasingly begun to feel as if she were unreal, in a dream, that "this couldn't really be me." She reports feeling "like a robot, just going through the motions." She feels very uncomfortable with these feelings. The latest and most frightening symptom was her sudden awareness that she could no longer "perceive colors." She feels that she can look at something and identify that it has a color but that she is seeing everything in shades of gray. Sue is worried that she is "going crazy." She says she is doing well at school and making friends.

Sue recently had her college-sports physical examination and was found to have no health problems. A psychosocial assessment reveals that this is Sue's first time away from home and that 4 months before she began college, her older brother was killed in an auto accident. The physician's preliminary diagnosis is depersonalization disorder.

Assessment *(nursing behaviors and rationales)*

1. Perform a health assessment and physical examination. *Physical problems must always be considered as a precipitant or cause of an apparent emotional problem. A thorough physical assessment and review of health history will reveal any such problems.*

2. Perform a psychosocial assessment. *A psychosocial assessment will help determine precipitating factors and the degree of impairment.*

3. Assess Sue's perception of the current problem. *The client's perceptions are the starting point for the nursing intervention. In this case, the client thought she was "going crazy," not connecting her symptoms with her two recent and significant losses (namely, her brother's death and her absence from home). A nursing assessment would bring out this knowledge deficit.*

Nursing diagnoses

- Anxiety related to the frightening symptoms
- Knowledge deficit related to inability to connect recent losses with stress and symptom formation
- Dysfunctional grieving related to leaving home and death of brother
- Personal identity disturbance related to feelings of being unreal
- Sensory-perceptual alterations (visual) related to inability to perceive color

Planning and goals

- Sue will be treated as an outpatient at the health center.
- Sue will experience reduced anxiety so that she can continue in her role performance and engage in psychotherapy.
- Sue will begin the healthy grieving process and learn effective coping skills.

Implementation *(nursing behaviors and rationales)*

1. Engage Sue in a therapeutic relationship. *This is the mechanism for achieving the goals related to anxiety reduction and achievement of healthy coping skills.*

2. Teach the client about the connection between severe stress levels and the development of psychological symptoms. *By making Sue aware that her severe losses may be an understandable precipitant to her feelings, she may feel less "crazy," stigmatized, and anxious.*

3. Encourage Sue to identify stressors and to develop healthy coping skills. *When Sue is able to see the symptoms as one potential outcome of her dysfunctional grieving, she will be less anxious and better able to be involved in her own care.*

4. Encourage Sue to continue to participate actively in campus life. *Such participation enables the client to develop new support systems while strengthening old ones.*

Evaluation

- Sue was able to finish her freshman year and improve her social life as she gradually felt "real" again.
- Sue became aware that the anniversary of her brother's death (toward the end of the semester) would be a stressful time; she made use of her newly strengthened support systems by expressing her feelings about his death.

13 Mood disorders

I. Overview

    A. Mood disorders, also known as affective disorders, are associated with a group of symptoms that result in severe and painful sadness or abnormal elation known clinically as a "high"

    B. These symptoms change a person's behavior, cognition, motivation, and emotions; in short, they change the person's physical, mental, and social being

    C. Mood disorders fall into one of two diagnostic categories

        1. In *major depression,* or *unipolar depression,* a person experiences one or more episodes of depression with no manic or hypomanic episode

            a. Major depression affects twice as many women as men

            b. Onset usually occurs in the person's middle thirties

            c. Major depression has a high prevalence among lower socioeconomic groups

        2. In *bipolar mood disorder,* a person experiences major depression with one or more manic or hypomanic episodes

            a. Bipolar disorder affects about the same number of men as women

            b. Onset usually occurs in the person's late twenties

            c. Bipolar disorder has a high prevalence among professional, well-educated groups

            d. Approximately 10% of those diagnosed with depression have a bipolar disorder

    D. Mood disorders vary in frequency, intensity, and duration

    E. They constitute the most common psychiatric diagnosis; about 5% of persons in the United States will have a mood disorder

II. Major depression (unipolar depression)

    A. Characteristics

        1. Anhedonia

        2. Sleep disturbances

        3. Loss of libido, appetite, energy, and interest

        4. Possible weight loss, fatigue, reduced cognition, and psychomotor agitation

5. Depression that may recur or consist of a single episode
6. Varied degree and intensity of symptoms

B. Types
1. *Agitated depression:* characterized by increased psychomotor activity
2. *Anxious depression:* characterized by prominent patterns of anxiety
3. *Atypical depression:* usually involves another condition, such as schizophrenia or dysthymic episode, besides the symptoms of depression
4. *Chronic depression:* lasts longer than 2 years; about 10% of those diagnosed with depression fall into this category
5. *Endogenous depression:* characterized by a biological cause, without known external stressors
6. *Involutional depression:* occurs in the person's late forties and fifties; women are more prone to involutional depression than men are
7. *Masked depression:* usually revealed during treatment of somatic complaints
8. *Paranoid depression:* characterized by paranoid ideation
9. *Postpartum depression:* can occur after childbirth, in three stages
   a. Within the first 3 to 4 days after delivery, the client may begin to feel "blue" and sad
   b. About the 3rd week after delivery, other symptoms of depression appear; these can last for about 1 year
   c. About 3 months after the delivery, confusion and disturbances in thought processes begin to accompany other symptoms
10. *Psychotic depression:* characterized by hallucinations or delusions
11. *Reactive depression:* associated with external stressors
12. *Retarded depression:* accompanied by decreased psychomotor activities
13. *Seasonal depression:* occurs during a specific season of the year

C. Theoretical perspectives
1. Biochemical theory
   a. Genetic markers have been found that substantiate a hereditary factor
   b. The blood levels of the biogenic amines norepinephrine, dopamine, and serotonin are deficient in people with depression
2. Psychodynamic theory
   a. Depression results from unresolved grieving in an early stage of the child-parent relationship
   b. The person remains fixed in the anger stage and turns the anger inward, toward the self, resulting in a weak ego and punitive superego

    3. Interpersonal theory

        a. The person is abandoned by or otherwise separated from the parent early in infancy (within the first 6 months), causing incomplete bonding, a predisposing factor

        b. Traumatic separation from a significant other in adulthood can be a precipitating factor; the person then withdraws from family and social contacts

    4. Behavioral theory

        a. Depression is believed to result from the interaction of the person-environment-behavior engagement

        b. The person has control over personal behavior but not over all environmental influences; consequently, the person may control some aspects of life but not be completely free to choose what happens in life

D. Diagnostic tests

    1. Dexamethasone-suppression test (DST): may be useful in diagnosing major depression

        a. In a nondepressed person, dexamethasone suppresses the production and release of cortisol from the adrenal gland

        b. In a depressed person, this suppression may be only partial, or the person may recover more rapidly from the dexamethasone effects

    2. Thyrotropin-releasing hormone (TRH) test: evaluates the ability of the pituitary to produce thyrotropin

E. Criteria for medical diagnosis (see the *DSM-III-R* diagnostic criteria for a major depressive episode on page 120)

F. Possible nursing diagnoses

    1. High risk for self-directed violence related to low self-esteem

    2. Ineffective individual coping related to guilt feelings

    3. Spiritual distress related to feelings of despair

    4. Sleep pattern disturbance related to desire to escape

    5. Impaired verbal communication related to lack of interest

G. General nursing interventions

    1. Identify the client's suicide potential

    2. Reevaluate the client's potential for suicide with any change in mood or behavior

    3. Create a safe environment

    4. Formulate a verbal contract with the client to notify staff members when feelings begin to get out of control

    5. Encourage the client to express anger in acceptable ways that are comfortable for the client

    6. Assist the client in recognizing strengths and accomplishments

    7. Teach effective communication skills

    8. Assist the client in performing activities of daily living

9. Provide positive reinforcement of acceptable behaviors
10. Assist the client in setting realistic goals
11. Help the client clarify thought processes
12. Discourage sleeping other than at bedtime
13. Teach relaxation techniques to use before bedtime
14. Limit time spent alone by encouraging participation in group activities
15. Provide simple activities that the client can successfully complete
16. Administer tricyclic antidepressants or monoamine oxidase (MAO) inhibitors, as prescribed

III. Bipolar disorder

A. Characteristics
1. Symptoms of major depression (see section II-A), accompanied by at least one episode of mania
2. Potential for psychotic features

B. Types
1. *Bipolar disorder, manic:* characterized by elation or irritability with excessive motor activity
2. *Bipolar disorder, mixed:* characterized by mood swings ranging from depression to euphoria, with intervening periods of normal behavior

C. Theoretical perspectives
1. Biological theory
    a. Genetic predisposition exists, especially if a female is diagnosed with the condition
    b. Increased levels of norepinephrine, a biogenic amine, appear in the brain of a manic client
2. Psychoanalytic theory
    a. Cyclic behaviors of depression and mania are responses to conditional love from the significant caregiver
    b. Ego development is disrupted because the child is in a dependent role, resulting in a punitive superego or a strong id

D. Criteria for medical diagnosis (see the *DSM-III-R* diagnostic criteria for bipolar disorder on pages 121 and 122)

E. Possible nursing diagnoses
1. High risk for injury related to agitation
2. Altered health maintenance related to hyperactivity
3. Sleep pattern disturbance related to restlessness
4. Self-care deficit related to inattention to personal needs
5. Impaired social interaction related to decreased attention span
6. Alteration in thought processes related to the psychotic process

(Text continues on page 122.)

Diagnostic criteria for mood disorders

The following chart presents the *DSM-III-R* diagnostic criteria for the mood disorders discussed in this chapter.

Major depressive episode

Note: A major depressive syndrome is defined as criterion A below.

A. At least five of the following nine symptoms must be present during the same 2-week period and must represent a change from a previous functioning level; at least one of the symptoms must be depressed mood or loss of interest or pleasure
   1. Depressed mood (or can be irritable mood in children and adolescents) most of the day, nearly every day, as indicated by the client's subjective reporting or observation by others
   2. Markedly diminished interest or pleasure in all, or almost all, activities most of the day, nearly every day (as indicated by the client's subjective reporting or observation by others of apathy most of the time)
   3. Significant weight loss or gain not attributable to diet (more than 5% change in body weight in a month) or decreased or increased appetite nearly every day (in children, consider failure to make expected weight gains as fitting this criterion)
   4. Insomnia or hypersomnia nearly every day
   5. Psychomotor agitation or retardation nearly every day (observable by others, not merely the client's subjective reporting of restlessness or feeling "slowed down")
   6. Fatigue or loss of energy nearly every day
   7. Feelings of worthlessness or excessive or inappropriate guilt (which may be delusional) nearly every day (not merely self-reproach or guilt about being sick)
   8. Indecisiveness or diminished ability to think or concentrate nearly every day (as indicated by the client's subjective reporting or observation by others)
   9. Recurrent thoughts of death (not just fear of dying), recurrent suicidal ideation, a specific plan for committing suicide, or a suicide attempt
B. It cannot be established that an organic factor initiated and maintained the depressive episode
C. The disturbance is not a normal reaction to the death of a loved one (uncomplicated bereavement)
D. At no time during the disturbance has the client experienced delusions or hallucinations in the absence of prominent mood symptoms (before the mood symptoms developed or after they have remitted)
E. The episode is not superimposed on schizophrenia, schizophreniform disorder, delusional disorder, or psychotic disorder not otherwise specified (NOS)
   Health care professionals use the following criteria to determine the severity of a major depressive episode.
Mild: few, if any, symptoms in excess of those required to make the diagnosis; symptoms result in only minor impairment in occupational functioning or in usual social activities or relationships with others
Moderate: symptoms of functional impairment that interfere with occupational, school, or social interactions

Diagnostic criteria for mood disorders *(continued)*

Severe, without psychotic features: several symptoms that exceed those required to make the diagnosis and that markedly interfere with occupational functioning or with usual social activities and relationships

Severe, with psychotic features: delusions or hallucinations that are either mood-congruent or mood-incongruent

- Mood-congruent psychotic features: delusions or hallucinations that are consistent with the typical depressive themes of personal inadequacy, guilt, disease, death, nihilism, or deserved punishment
- Mood-incongruent psychotic features: delusions or hallucinations *not* involving the typical depressive themes stated above (such as persecutory delusions, thought insertion, thought broadcasting, and delusions of control)

Manic episode

Note: A manic syndrome is defined as including criteria A, B, and C below; a hypomanic syndrome is defined as including criteria A and B, but not C (that is, no marked impairment).

A. The person experiences a distinct period of abnormally and persistently elevated, expansive, or irritable mood

B. During the period of mood disturbance, at least three of the following symptoms have persisted (four if the mood is only irritable) and have been present to a significant degree
   1. Inflated self-esteem or grandiosity
   2. Decreased need for sleep (the client feels rested after only 3 hours of sleep)
   3. Tendency to talk more than usual or to feel pressured to keep talking
   4. Flight of ideas or a subjective experience that thoughts are racing
   5. Distractibility, attention too easily drawn to unimportant or irrelevant external stimuli
   6. Increase in goal-directed activity (in social situations, at work, in school, or in sexual relations) or psychomotor agitation
   7. Excessive involvement in pleasurable activities that have a high potential for painful consequences (for example, the client engages in unrestrained buying sprees, sexual indiscretions, or foolish business investments)

C. The mood disturbance is sufficiently severe to cause marked impairment in occupational functioning, usual social activities, or relationships with others or to necessitate hospitalization to prevent harm to self or others

D. At no time during the manic episode has the person experienced delusions or hallucinations for as long as 2 weeks in the absence of prominent mood symptoms (that is, before the mood symptoms developed or after they remitted)

E. The disturbance is not superimposed on schizophrenia, schizophreniform disorder, delusional disorder, or psychotic disorder not otherwise specified (NOS)

F. It cannot be established that an organic factor initiated and maintained the manic episode (somatic antidepressant treatments, such as drugs and electroconvulsive therapy, that appear to precipitate a mood disturbance should not be considered a causative organic factor)

Health care professionals use the following criteria to determine the severity of a manic episode.

Mild: meets minimum symptom criteria for a manic episode

Moderate: extreme increase in activity or impairment in judgment

(continued)

Diagnostic criteria for mood disorders *(continued)*

Severe, without psychotic features: psychomotor activity so extreme as to require almost continual supervision in order to prevent physical harm to the client or others

Severe, with psychotic features: delusions, hallucinations, or catatonic symptoms that are either mood-congruent or mood-incongruent

• Mood-congruent psychotic features: delusions or hallucinations that are consistent with the typical manic themes of inflated worth, power, knowledge, identity, or special relationship to a deity or famous person

• Mood-incongruent psychotic features: catatonic symptoms (such as stupor, mutism, negativism, or posturing) or delusions or hallucinations *not* involving the typical manic themes stated above (such as persecutory delusions, thought insertion, and delusions of being controlled)

Source: *Diagnostic and Statistical Manual of Mental Disorders,* Third Edition-Revised. Washington, D.C.: American Psychiatric Association, 1987. Adapted with permission.

F. General nursing interventions
  1. Reduce environmental stimuli
  2. Limit the client's participation in group activities
  3. Create a safe environment
  4. Provide physical exercise as a substitute for increased motor activity
  5. Avoid arguments or confrontations with the client
  6. Instruct the client on using more socially appropriate behaviors
  7. Provide positive feedback for socially acceptable behaviors
  8. Monitor eating and sleeping patterns
  9. Restrict caffeine intake
  10. Limit the selection of clothing available
  11. Set goals for minimal standards of personal hygiene
  12. Keep the client oriented to reality
  13. Assist the client in focusing on a single task
  14. Limit invasion of the client's personal space by other clients and staff
  15. Encourage rest periods
  16. Administer lithium, tranquilizers, or antipsychotics, as prescribed

Clinical situation

Mary Boggs, age 36, is admitted to the inpatient psychiatric treatment facility of a local hospital with a tentative diagnosis of major depression. She has just been treated in the emergency department for attempting suicide by taking 20 tablets of Xanax 10 mg. About 3 months ago, her boyfriend broke off his relationship with Mary to pursue another woman. Since that time, Mary has been put on probation at work because of many absences and her inability to complete work assignments.

Mary states that she has trouble sleeping and has not been able to concentrate. Finding no humor in life, she dreads getting out of bed in the morning to face the world, and she has stopped socializing with her girlfriends. Mary says she has never felt this bad before and can't seem to get her life together. She feels worthless; she apologizes to you for her lack of personal hygiene, saying that she was never like this before.

Mary states that she had lived with her boyfriend for 6 years; when they broke up, she had to move back home because of inadequate finances. Since then, her parents have told her that she will never amount to anything.

Assessment *(nursing behaviors and rationales)*

1. Perform a physical assessment, noting any somatic complaints, changes in eating and sleeping patterns, and level of concentration. *Physical problems (such as tumors, infections, endocrine disorders, anemia, and electrolyte imbalances) can produce depressive symptoms.*

2. Assess whether Mary can meet self-care needs satisfactorily. *Performing activities of daily living may be difficult for a depressed person, whose energy level typically decreases. Failure to meet self-care needs leads to feelings of hopelessness and unworthiness.*

3. Assess Mary's potential for suicide; determine if she is currently suicidal. *Clients with a history of previous suicide attempts, and those who are depressed, are at higher risk for attempting suicide than are clients with no previous history or no depressive symptoms. Clients whose depression is lifting are at higher risk of suicide than those severely depressed because they now have the energy, as the depression lifts, to commit suicide.*

4. Perform a psychosocial assessment, inquiring about social interaction and coping patterns, life stressors, and previous experiences with sadness. *Having the client explain previous behaviors will assist the nurse in determining the severity and duration of the current depression.*

5. Assess the client's perception of the situation. *Distorted perceptions about what is happening is a symptom of depression. Changes in perceptions suggest changes in the depressed state.*

Nursing diagnoses
- High risk for self-directed violence related to despair
- Ineffective individual coping related to anxiety
- Self-esteem disturbance related to feelings of worthlessness
- Social isolation related to withdrawn behavior
- Sleep pattern disturbance related to worrying

Planning and goals
- Mary Boggs will remain safe from suicidal impulses.
- She will perform activities of daily living, such as personal hygiene, independently.
- She will speak positively about her appearance and accomplishments.
- She will be able to sleep at least 6 hours nightly by the time of discharge.

Implementation *(nursing behaviors and rationales)*

1. Monitor Mary's potential for suicide by directly asking her if she is suicidal. *Clients who have attempted suicide are at higher risk than those who have not.*

Most people who state an intention to commit suicide ultimately succeed unless someone intervenes. Psychotic thoughts add to the suicide risk.

2. Place Mary on suicidal observation, if indicated. Explain that you want to keep Mary safe until she can keep herself safe. *In an unsafe environment, suicidal people are more likely to attempt suicide impulsively. The nurse's caring attitude may give the client a sense of protection. Suicide precautions (including monitoring the client's whereabouts, bathroom use, use of personal-care items, and taking of medication) provide safety for the client.*

3. Secure a promise from Mary that she will talk to a staff member if suicidal thoughts emerge. *Suicidal clients require a safe, secure environment, along with staff members who will be there to prevent a suicide attempt, if necessary. Having someone to talk with may reduce the client's anxiety.*

4. Encourage Mary to verbalize her feelings about her previous romantic relationship. *Talking about these feelings may help the client begin to deal more effectively with the loss.*

5. Have Mary describe what happened at work and home before she came to the hospital. *This helps the client see her problems from a different perspective. By learning to consider all aspects of a situation, the client is developing an effective coping strategy.*

6. Promote the development of Mary's social and leisure skills. *This will help Mary regain self-confidence and will assist in reducing her social isolation.*

7. Involve Mary in physical exercise and play activities. *These activities release tension and promote the development of new coping skills.*

8. Assist Mary in identifying people she can ask for help after being discharged. *Having a support system decreases feelings of despair and reduces the likelihood of future suicide attempts.*

9. Teach Mary and her family about depressive behavior. *The client and her family probably do not understand that her behavior is the result of an illness. Knowledge about depression will help the client deal more effectively with her behavior and will enable her family to be more supportive during her postdischarge treatment.*

Evaluation

- Mary makes no further attempts at suicide.
- Mary attends to her activities of daily living without assistance.
- Mary sleeps a minimum of 6 hours at night.
- Mary participates in social activities with other clients and staff.
- Mary sets realistic goals for her work and living arrangements.
- Mary develops a support system of family and friends.

14 Organic mental syndromes

I. Overview

A. An organic mental syndrome is a mental disorder whose cause is known or can be reasonably presumed

B. An essential feature of the condition is a psychological or behavioral abnormality associated with transient or permanent brain dysfunction

C. Organic mental syndromes are heterogeneous
  1. No single description can aptly characterize them all
  2. They differ in clinical presentation, location, mode of onset, progression, duration, and nature of the underlying pathophysiologic process

D. Predisposing factors include chronic physical illness, alcohol dependence, death of a close friend or family member (including a pet), marital separation, or a natural disaster

E. The most common organic mental syndromes are associated with Axis III physical disorders; they include delirium, dementia, amnestic syndrome, organic hallucinosis, and organic personality syndrome

II. Delirium

A. Characteristics
  1. Acute brain dysfunction marked by a deficiency in the capacity to maintain attention
  2. Result of various physical causes, including infection, an endocrine disorder, trauma, or drug abuse
  3. Rapid onset (within hours or days) and usually brief duration
  4. Varying course of illness that depends on identifying and correcting the causative agent

B. Signs and symptoms
  1. Disorganized thought processes
  2. Apathy
  3. Clouded sensorium
  4. Impaired cognition
  5. Decreased level of consciousness
  6. Disorientation
  7. Disturbances in perception

C. Criteria for medical diagnosis (see the *DSM-III-R* diagnostic criteria for delirium on page 129)

D. Possible nursing diagnoses
  1. Altered thought processes related to changes in brain function
  2. Impaired verbal communication related to incoherent speech
  3. Self-care deficit related to inability to perform activities of daily living
  4. Sensory-perceptual alteration related to disorientation

E. General nursing interventions
  1. Keep the client oriented to reality
    a. Call the client by name
    b. Keep a clock and calendar in plain view
  2. Use simple words and short sentences to communicate
  3. Assist the client with personal hygiene; establish a routine for dressing
  4. Provide a safe, quiet environment

III. Dementia

A. Characteristics
  1. Memory impairment and insidious loss of intellectual ability
  2. Varying onset; may be rapid (such as from head trauma) or slow (such as from Alzheimer's disease)
  3. Progressive, static, or recurring course, depending on pathogenesis
  4. Prevalence among elderly clients (but can occur in any age-group)

B. Signs and symptoms
  1. Short- and long-term memory impairment
  2. Premorbid personality changes
  3. Disturbed judgment
  4. Difficulty in understanding the meaning of words
  5. Confusion
  6. Depressed affect

C. Criteria for medical diagnosis (see the *DSM-III-R* diagnostic criteria for dementia on pages 129 and 130)

D. Possible nursing diagnoses
  1. Altered thought processes related to inaccurate interpretation of environmental stimuli
  2. Altered nutrition (less than body requirements) related to failure to remember mealtimes
  3. High risk for injury related to disorientation and confusion
  4. Ineffective family coping (compromised) related to family's inability to deal with changes in the client's personality

E. General nursing interventions
1. Keep the client oriented to reality
2. Label furniture, rooms, and clothing
3. Speak slowly, and repeat instructions several times
4. Provide a safe environment
5. Frequently monitor the client's whereabouts
6. Put the client on a consistent meal schedule; observe the client's food intake
7. Teach the client's family about the disease and how they can adjust to changes in the client's behavior

IV. Amnestic syndrome

A. Characteristics
1. Short- and long-term memory impairment without clouding of consciousness or intellectual deterioration
2. Result of a specific organic insult to the brain
   a. Anterograde memory loss (the client cannot remember events that occurred after the brain insult)
   b. Retrograde memory loss (the client cannot remember events that occurred before the brain insult)
3. Confabulation commonly used as a defense mechanism

B. Signs and symptoms
1. Inability to recall recent events
2. Inability to retain newly learned material
3. Observable or laboratory test evidence of organic brain insult (such as from trauma or a vitamin deficiency)

C. Criteria for medical diagnosis (see the *DSM-III-R* diagnostic criteria for amnestic syndrome on page 130)

D. Possible nursing diagnoses
1. Altered nutrition (less than body requirements) related to a nutrient deficiency
2. Impaired adjustment related to memory loss
3. High risk for injury related to inability to learn safety rules
4. Ineffective family coping (compromised) related to poor family adjustment to the client's behavior

E. General nursing interventions
1. Monitor the client's food and fluid intake
2. Supervise the client's travel away from home
3. Establish a training program for relearning information needed to exist safely in the environment
4. Institute memory therapy (for example, by teaching mnemonics)
5. Teach the family coping techniques and ways to meet the client's safety needs

V. Organic hallucinosis

A. Characteristics
  1. Persistent and recurring hallucinations that have a specific organic cause (the client may or may not believe the hallucinations are real)
  2. Varying forms of hallucinations, depending on the underlying cause
    a. Auditory hallucinations from such conditions as otosclerosis
    b. Visual hallucinations from such conditions as hallucinogen abuse

B. Signs and symptoms
  1. Persistent and recurring hallucinations
  2. Observable or laboratory test evidence of an organic cause

C. Criteria for medical diagnosis (see the *DSM-III-R* diagnostic criteria for organic hallucinosis on page 130)

D. Possible nursing diagnoses
  1. High risk for injury related to the client's attempts to escape from the hallucinations
  2. Altered thought processes related to the hallucinations
  3. Sleep disturbances related to the hallucinations
  4. Sensory-perceptual alterations (visual, auditory, kinesthetic, gustatory, tactile, olfactory) related to alcohol or drug intake

E. General nursing interventions
  1. Provide a protective environment for the client
  2. Provide structured recreational activities and a routine for activities of daily living
  3. Give accurate information to the client about the hallucinations
  4. Reassure the client that hallucinations are not a sign that the client is having a mental breakdown

VI. Organic personality syndrome

A. Characteristics
  1. Emotional lability
  2. Evidence of an organic factor that preceded and is related to the personality change
  3. Outcome dependent on the underlying cause
    a. May be reversible if the cause is chronic intoxication
    b. May remain static if the cause is frontal lobe trauma

B. Signs and symptoms
  1. Recurrent outbursts of hostile, aggressive behavior
  2. Apathy and indifference
  3. Dramatic mood shifts (from stable mood to depression to irritability)
  4. Poor impulse control (for example, commission of sexual indiscretions)

Diagnostic criteria for organic mental syndromes

The following chart presents the *DSM-III-R* diagnostic criteria for the organic mental syndromes discussed in this chapter.

Delirium
A. The person has a reduced ability to maintain attention to external stimuli (for example, questions must be repeated because the person's attention wanders) and to shift attention appropriately to new external stimuli (for example, the person continues to repeat the answer to a previous question)

B. The person exhibits disorganized thinking, as indicated by rambling, irrelevant, or incoherent speech

C. The person experiences at least two of the following:
  1. Reduced level of consciousness (such as difficulty keeping awake during the examination)
  2. Perceptual disturbances: misinterpretations, illusions, or hallucinations
  3. Disturbance of sleep-wake cycle with insomnia or daytime sleepiness
  4. Increased or decreased psychomotor activity
  5. Disorientation to time, place, or person
  6. Memory impairment (for instance, an inability to learn new material, such as the names of several unrelated objects after 5 minutes, or to remember past events, such as the history of the current episode of illness)

D. Clinical features develop over a short period (usually hours to days) and tend to fluctuate over the course of the day

E. The disturbance meets either of the following criteria:
  1. The history, physical examination, or laboratory tests show evidence of one or more specific organic factors judged to be etiologically related to the disturbance
  2. The disturbance cannot be accounted for by any nonorganic mental disorder (such as a manic episode accounting for agitation and sleep disturbance)

Dementia
A. The person shows demonstrable evidence of short- and long-term memory impairment
  1. Short-term memory impairment (inability to learn new information) may be indicated by an inability to remember three objects after five minutes
  2. Long-term memory impairment (inability to remember information previously known) may be indicated by an inability to remember personal information (such as one's birthplace or occupation) or facts of common knowledge (such as past U.S. presidents or well-known historical dates)

B. The person exhibits at least one of the following:
  1. Impairment in abstract thinking, as indicated by an inability to find similarities and differences between related words, difficulty in defining words and concepts, and other similar tasks
  2. Impaired judgment, as indicated by an inability to make reasonable plans to deal with interpersonal, family, and job-related problems and issues

(continued)

Diagnostic criteria for organic mental syndromes *(continued)*

3. Other disturbances of higher cortical function, such as aphasia (disorder of language), apraxia (inability to carry out motor activities despite intact comprehension and motorfunction), agnosia (failure to recognize or identify objects despite intact sensory function), and "constructional difficulty" (for example, an inability to copy three-dimensional figures, assemble blocks, or arrange sticks in specific designs)
4. Personality change (that is, an alteration or accentuation of premorbid traits)

C. The disturbance in A and B significantly interferes with the person's work or usual social activities or relationships with others

D. The disturbance does not occur exclusively during the course of delirium

E. The disturbance meets either of the following criteria:
1. The history, physical examination, or laboratory tests show evidence of one or more specific organic factors judged to be etiologically related to the disturbance
2. The disturbance cannot be accounted for by any nonorganic mental disorder (such as major depression accounting for cognitive impairment)

Health care professionals use the following criteria to determine the severity of dementia.
Mild: Although work or social activities are significantly impaired, the capacity for independent living remains, with adequate personal hygiene and relatively intact judgment
Moderate: Independent living is hazardous, and some degree of supervision is necessary
Severe: Activities of daily living are so impaired that continual supervision is required (for instance, the person cannot maintain minimal personal hygiene or is largely incoherent or mute)

Amnestic syndrome

A. The person shows demonstrable evidence of short- and long-term memory impairment
1. Short-term memory impairment (inability to learn new information) may be indicated by an inability to remember three objects after five minutes
2. Long-term memory impairment (inability to remember information previously known) may be indicated by an inability to remember personal information (such as one's birthplace or occupation) or facts of common knowledge (such as past U.S. presidents or well-known historical dates); the person remembers extremely remote events better than more recent events

B. The disturbance does not occur exclusively during the course of delirium and does not meet the criteria for dementia (that is, the person shows no impairment in abstract thinking or judgment, no other disturbances of higher cortical function, and no personality change)

C. The history, physical examination, or laboratory tests show evidence of one or more specific organic factors judged to be etiologically related to the disturbance

Organic hallucinosis

A. The person experiences prominent persistent or recurrent hallucinations

B. The history, physical examination, or laboratory tests show evidence of one or more specific organic factors judged to be etiologically related to the disturbance

C. The disturbance does not occur exclusively during the course of delirium

Diagnostic criteria for organic mental syndromes *(continued)*

Organic personality syndrome

A. The person exhibits a persistent personality disturbance (either lifelong or representing a change from or accentuation of a previously characteristic trait) involving at least one of the following:

  1. Affective instability (such as marked shifts from normal mood to depression, irritability, or anxiety)

  2. Recurrent outbursts of aggression or rage that are grossly out of proportion to any precipitating psychosocial stressors

  3. Markedly impaired social judgment (for instance, as indicated by sexual indiscretions)

  4. Marked apathy and indifference

  5. Suspiciousness or paranoid ideation

B. The history, physical examination, or laboratory tests show evidence of one or more specific organic factors judged to be etiologically related to the disturbance

C. The person is not a child or adolescent whose clinical status is limited to the features that characterize attention-deficit hyperactivity disorder

D. The disturbance does not occur exclusively during the course of delirium and does not meet the criteria for dementia

Source: *Diagnostic and Statistical Manual of Mental Disorders*, Third Edition-Revised. Washington, D.C.: American Psychiatric Association, 1987. Adapted with permission.

C. Criteria for medical diagnosis (see the *DSM-III-R* diagnostic criteria for organic personality syndrome in the chart above)

D. Possible nursing diagnoses

  1. Impaired social interaction related to outbursts of aggression

  2. Noncompliance with the treatment plan related to hostility

  3. High risk for violence directed at others related to poor impulse control

E. General nursing interventions

  1. Enforce behavioral limits and standards consistently

  2. Discuss the client's behavior in a nonjudgmental way

  3. Encourage the client to talk about feelings

  4. Manage the client's physical aggression immediately and safely with medication or seclusion, as needed

  5. Involve the client as much as possible in decisions affecting care

Clinical situation Charles Ames, age 78, was recently treated for abdominal pain in an acute-care facility. Although the course of treatment was uneventful, Mr. Ames became confused and disoriented during hospitalization. He sometimes misidentified family members when they came to visit. He would wander the halls at night, entering other clients' rooms and going through their personal belongings. Attempts at restraining him were unsuccessful; he would fight the staff, kick, yell, and create a disturbance on the unit. Because of this behavior, the physician prescribed 5 mg of haloperidol (Haldol) every 4 hours, as needed.

Two days ago, Mr. Ames wandered out of the hospital and had to be picked up by the police. On his return, his appetite decreased. He became easily frustrated and, on one occasion, threw his bath water at the nurse.

Today he is being admitted to your long-term-care facility with a diagnosis of primary degenerative dementia. You note that he appears angry, frightened, disoriented, and sedated. Very frail, Mr. Ames needs assistance to sit in a chair.

Assessment *(nursing behaviors and rationales)*

1. Perform a physical assessment. *Because the client has a recent history of not eating, he may be undernourished, and this would need to be corrected. Additionally, the client may have sustained injuries while wandering away from the hospital.*

2. Assess the client's orientation to time, place, and person. *The client may become more confused and disoriented on transferring to a new facility.*

3. Assess behavioral and personality changes in Mr. Ames. *Ritualistic behavior may be present. Wandering or hostility toward attempts at controlling the client will require intervention.*

4. Assess the client's ability to perform self-care. *Disorganization, forgetfulness, and motor impairment may reduce the client's ability to perform activities of daily living independently.*

5. Assess for cognitive impairment in Mr. Ames. *The nurse must determine whether the client shows evidence of cognitive impairment (such as loss of problem-solving ability) in order to establish which functions the client can carry out independently.*

Nursing diagnoses

• High risk for injury related to inability to recognize and identify dangers in the environment
• Altered thought processes related to memory loss
• Sensory-perceptual alteration related to irreversible neuron degeneration
• Sleep pattern disturbance related to disorientation (day-night reversal)
• Personal identity disturbance related to brain function alteration and to relocation to the long-term-care facility
• Self-care deficit related to cognitive decline
• Altered nutrition (less than body requirements) related to loss of appetite

Planning and goals

• Mr. Ames will no longer wander away.
• Mr. Ames will retire at an established time each night and will sleep for at least 6 hours.
• Mr. Ames's appetite will return, and he will eat three nutritious meals a day.
• Mr. Ames's agitation will diminish.

Implementation (nursing behaviors and rationales)

1. Call Mr. Ames by name at least four times each shift. *Calling the client by name helps the client retain his individuality and maintain his orientation, thereby reducing confusion and agitation.*

2. Do not permit Mr. Ames to sleep during the day. Provide regular social activities and exercise periods during waking hours. *Sleeping during the day can contribute to wakefulness at night. Daily activities and exercise promote a more restful nighttime sleep.*

3. Mark Mr. Ames's room and public areas with signs so that he can become familiar with his surroundings. *A recently transferred client, especially one with dementia, can easily become confused by a new environment. Helping the client adjust to his new surroundings may reduce agitation, confusion, and wandering behavior.*

4. Provide Mr. Ames with small nourishing meals, including puddings, juice, and fortified liquids. Provide a quiet place for him to eat. *Small meals will help promote an increased appetite. Fortified liquids will reestablish the client's nutritional balance. A quiet place can help minimize or prevent distraction from eating.*

5. Closely monitor Mr. Ames's physical mobility while allowing as much independent movement as he can safely accomplish. *The client's frailty may cause him to fall. Knowing which activities the client can safely perform — and always monitoring his whereabouts — will enable the nurse to prevent the client from wandering or causing self-harm. Independence is important to maintain the client's self-esteem.*

6. Speak to Mr. Ames in a soft, clear, unhurried manner. *A pleasant voice helps promote client comprehension and poses no threat to the client. Conversely, loud, hurried speech from the nurse can convey stress and anger, which may trigger memories of unpleasant experiences and result in an angry response from the client.*

7. Monitor Mr. Ames's laboratory test results for adverse effects of medication, including signs of overdose. *The client may have built up toxic serum drug levels with long-term use. If so, the physician may need to reduce the dosage.*

8. Offer clothing items, one at a time, as Mr. Ames dresses. Tell him how to put on each garment. *Simplicity reduces frustration and the potential for agitation and despair. Coaching reduces confusion.*

Evaluation

- Mr. Ames knows how to get to and from the day room and bathroom without getting lost.
- Mr. Ames responds to people in his environment and answers when called by name.
- Mr. Ames sleeps 6 to 8 hours every night without waking and wandering.
- Mr. Ames successfully performs activities of daily living with minimal supervision or assistance.
- Mr. Ames adheres to an individualized meal plan that includes many of his food preferences, and his appetite returns.

15 Personality disorders

I. Overview

A. On a social response continuum, interpersonal relationships range from adaptive behaviors to maladaptive ones
   1. Adaptive behaviors provide for mutually satisfying interactions
   2. Maladaptive behaviors result in loneliness, suspiciousness, and withdrawn behavior

B. Personality disorders fall somewhere within the maladaptive range; the degree of maladaptation depends on the type of disorder and the severity of symptoms

C. The behavioral responses of an individual with a personality disorder are inflexible
   1. The behaviors cause marked social impairment and disruption in vocational functioning; in short, they render the individual incapable of functioning effectively in society
   2. The individual remains totally unaware of these adverse impacts
   3. The individual reacts to stress and anxiety by trying to change the surrounding environment
   4. The individual perceives character flaws not only as acceptable and unobjectionable to others but also as positive aspects of the individual's character
   5. The individual does not accept blame for hurting someone

D. The *DSM-III-R* classifies personality disorders as Axis II diagnoses that fall into one of three clusters
   1. Cluster A consists of paranoid, schizoid, and schizotypal personality disorders
      a. An individual with one of these disorders is aloof and emotionally distant from others
      b. The person's behaviors are considered strange or eccentric
   2. Cluster B consists of antisocial, borderline, histrionic, and narcissistic personality disorders
      a. An individual with one of these disorders appears extremely egocentric, with little ability to understand another's perspective
      b. The person's behaviors are erratic and dramatic

    3. Cluster C consists of avoidant, dependent, obsessive-compulsive, and passive-aggressive personality disorders

        a. An individual with one of these disorders appears overly anxious about various social and personal issues

        b. The person tends to be unusually concerned with rules, procedures, and acceptance by others

II. Theoretical perspectives

A. Biological theory

    1. A genetic predisposition to personality disorders exists, especially among individuals with a cluster A disorder or those with a family history of alcoholism or other psychiatric problem

    2. An individual with schizoid personality disorder, for example, is likely to have a family member who is schizophrenic

B. Psychodynamic theory

    1. Poor parenting during the first 5 years of life results in inadequate mastery of developmental issues and conflicts centering on autonomy, separation-individuation, abandonment, dependency, control, or authority

    2. Individuals who had a cold, indifferent, and emotionally deficient childhood have a good chance of developing a personality disorder

C. Sociocultural theory

    1. In some cultures, gender-specific child-rearing practices may predispose women to dependent personality disorder

    2. Cultural norms influence the establishment of relationships; casual friendships may not be encouraged

    3. Social mobility and lack of close family ties promote loneliness and involuntary isolation

III. Paranoid personality disorder

A. Characteristics

    1. Suspiciousness

    2. Conviction that other people "are out to do me in"

    3. Inability to discern the context of a given situation, so that the person misperceives single acts or events within the situation

    4. Cold, aloof, overly serious affect

    5. Inability to experience or express warmth and tenderness

    6. Use of projection as a primary defense mechanism

B. Criteria for medical diagnosis (see the *DSM-III-R* diagnostic criteria for paranoid personality disorder on page 142)

C. Treatment

    1. Neuroleptic therapy

    2. Symptom management

        3. *Note:* Therapies involving confrontation of feelings and alliances with others are *not* effective

    D. Possible nursing diagnoses

        1. Altered growth and development related to unmet childhood needs

        2. Altered parenting related to lack of knowledge about the parenting role

        3. High risk for violence directed at others related to antisocial character

        4. Fear related to being harmed by others

    E. General nursing interventions

        1. Maintain an unambiguous environment

        2. Clarify the meanings and contexts of conversations, situations, and events

        3. Develop and nurture trust in the nurse-client relationship

IV. Schizoid personality disorder

    A. Characteristics

        1. Steadfast determination to remain distant and aloof

        2. Preference for solitary activities to those requiring interaction with others

        3. Inability to form relationships, impoverished social skills, lack of desire to develop social contacts

        4. Emotionally restricted affect; rare (if any) expression of feelings

        5. Use of intellectualization as a primary defense mechanism

    B. Criteria for medical diagnosis (see the *DSM-III-R* diagnostic criteria for schizoid personality disorder on page 142)

    C. Treatment: outpatient therapies designed to increase interpersonal comfort

    D. Possible nursing diagnoses

        1. Diversional activity deficit related to unsustained social contact

        2. Social isolation related to aloof, withdrawn behavior

    E. General nursing interventions

        1. Provide safety in the nurse-client interaction

        2. Allow the physical and emotional space needed by the client

        3. Foster the development of basic social skills (providing for the client's daily needs should supercede diversional activity)

V. Schizotypal personality disorder

    A. Characteristics

        1. Eccentric behavior

        2. Expression of unusual ideas

        3. Magical thinking (belief that the individual possesses special powers)

      4. Inability to form and maintain age-appropriate relationships

      5. Anxiety in social situations

      6. Dysphoria

B. Criteria for medical diagnosis (see the *DSM-III-R* diagnostic criteria for schizotypal personality disorder on pages 142 and 143)

C. Treatment

      1. Neuroleptic therapy

      2. Social skills development

      3. Guidance in the management of daily affairs

      4. *Note:* Intensive psychotherapy generally is *not* effective

D. Possible nursing diagnoses

      1. Altered role performance related to eccentric behavior

      2. Altered thought processes related to odd ideas

      3. Self-care deficit related to inability to take care of personal affairs

      4. Sensory-perceptual alteration related to self-centered feelings

E. General nursing interventions

      1. Institute safety precautions

      2. Assist the client in developing rudimentary social skills

      3. Help the client with personal grooming and hygiene

VI. Antisocial personality disorder

A. Characteristics

      1. Consistent antisocial behavior (more common in males)

      2. Sustained history of irresponsibility and impulsiveness

      3. Lack of remorse for one's destructive actions

      4. Manipulation and exploitation of others

      5. Extreme self-centeredness

      6. Belief that one's actions are justified

      7. Anxiety and depression

      8. Anger that results in hostile outbursts

      9. Use of rationalization and acting out as primary defense mechanisms

B. Criteria for medical diagnosis (see the *DSM-III-R* diagnostic criteria for antisocial personality disorder on pages 143 and 144)

C. Treatment

      1. Group psychotherapy

      2. Confrontation of inappropriate behaviors

D. Possible nursing diagnoses

      1. Noncompliance with treatment related to the client's denial of problems

      2. High risk for violence related to a disregard for the feelings of others

        3. Sexual dysfunction related to harmful relationships

        4. Impaired social interactions related to a disregard for the feelings or property of others

  E. General nursing interventions

        1. Provide a stable environment

        2. Apply behavioral limits judiciously

        3. Assist the client in taking responsibility for the consequences of actions

VII. Borderline personality disorder

  A. Characteristics

        1. Impulsiveness

        2. Outbursts of intense anger and rage

        3. Emotional lability

        4. Unstable identity

        5. Inability to be alone

        6. Self-mutilation

        7. Harmful, unstable, intense relationships

        8. Bouts of depression

        9. Anxiety

      10. Use of splitting, idealization, devaluation, and projective identification as primary defense mechanisms

  B. Criteria for medical diagnosis (see the *DSM-III-R* diagnostic criteria for borderline personality disorder on pages 144 and 145)

  C. Treatment

        1. Group psychotherapy

        2. Individual psychotherapy

        3. Structured living under supervision

        4. Neuroleptic therapy

  D. Possible nursing diagnoses

        1. Ineffective individual coping related to unmet dependency needs

        2. Self-esteem disturbance related to feelings of worthlessness

        3. Personal identity disturbance related to identity uncertainty

        4. High risk for self-directed violence related to manipulative behavior

  E. General nursing interventions

        1. Provide a structured, supportive, and consistent environment

        2. Counter the client's attempts to cause dissension among staff members

           a. Adhere strictly to the treatment plan

           b. Refuse to engage in third-party conversations

VIII. Histrionic personality disorder

    A. Characteristics

        1. Melodramatic, colorful, highly energetic personality

        2. Development of shallow relationships

        3. Tendency to make many demands upon others for reassurance

        4. Somatic complaints, marked by exaggeration of symptoms

        5. Seductive, self-centered nature

        6. Inability to establish genuinely intimate relationships

        7. Bursts of exaggerated emotion in any situation

        8. Use of somatization and dissociation as primary defense mechanisms

    B. Criteria for medical diagnosis (see the *DSM-III-R* diagnostic criteria for histrionic personality disorder on page 145)

    C. Treatment: outpatient supportive therapy

    D. Possible nursing diagnoses

        1. Self-esteem disturbance related to unsatisfactory personal relationships

        2. Impaired social interaction related to seductive behavior

        3. High risk for violence related to poor impulse control

    E. General nursing interventions

        1. Allay the client's anxiety about meeting needs for love and affection

        2. Teach the client ways to delay needs for gratification

        3. Assist the client in assuming a mature adult role

        4. Assist the client in identifying feelings and in learning how to express them in a socially acceptable manner

IX. Narcissistic personality disorder

    A. Characteristics

        1. Inflated sense of self-importance

        2. Feelings of entitlement to recognition

        3. Craving and search for constant attention

        4. Feelings of worthlessness if not lavishly praised and admired by others

        5. Development of shallow interpersonal relationships based primarily on how others can meet the client's needs for esteem

        6. Complete lack of empathy

        7. Depression

        8. Rage

        9. Shame and humiliation

      10. Use of idealization as a primary defense mechanism

    B. Criteria for medical diagnosis (see the *DSM-III-R* diagnostic criteria for narcissistic personality disorder on pages 145 and 146)

C. Treatment: individual or group therapy

D. Possible nursing diagnoses
1. Self-esteem disturbance related to feelings of worthlessness
2. Altered role performance related to demands for attention
3. Defensive coping related to grandiosity

E. General nursing interventions
1. Enhance the client's self-esteem and sense of self-worth
2. Assist the client in identifying feelings and in learning how to express them in a socially acceptable manner
3. Maintain a stable environment for the client, and apply limits consistently
   a. These interventions tend to enhance the individual's sense of safety
   b. They also can help reduce manipulative behaviors

X. Avoidant personality disorder

A. Characteristics
1. Avoidance of any situation that could result in criticism
2. Hypersensitivity to rejection
3. Ineptitude and discomfort in social settings (social phobias may be evident), despite craving the interpersonal contacts the client so fearfully shuns
4. Anxiety and depression
5. Anger
6. Use of avoidance as a primary defense mechanism

B. Criteria for medical diagnosis (see the *DSM-III-R* diagnostic criteria for avoidant personality disorder on page 146)

C. Treatment
1. Assertiveness training
2. Social skills training
3. Relaxation exercises

D. Possible nursing diagnoses
1. Social isolation related to shunning interpersonal contact
2. Anxiety related to the possibility of making social mistakes
3. Powerlessness related to helpless life-style
4. Self-esteem disturbance related to feelings of being unable to deal with life's events

E. General nursing interventions
1. Enhance the individual's ability to confront social situations
2. Role-play events; then discuss what the client thought would happen

XI. Dependent personality disorder

A. Characteristics
1. Unassertiveness and passivity
2. Abdication of decision making to others
3. Belief that one will not be liked or will be abandoned if one offends another
4. Inability to take risks or to initiate anything without prior approval from others
5. Depression and anxiety
6. Use of self-devaluation as a defense mechanism

B. Criteria for medical diagnosis (see the *DSM-III-R* diagnostic criteria for dependent personality disorder on page 146)

C. Treatment
1. Assertiveness training
2. Relaxation exercises

D. Possible nursing diagnoses
1. Impaired adjustment related to dependence on others
2. Decisional conflict (delayed decision making) related to lack of experience in making choices without help
3. Altered role performance related to fear of initiating actions

E. General nursing interventions
1. Enhance the client's ability to speak up and assume age-appropriate responsibilities
2. Give assignments that involve the client in risk-taking behaviors

XII. Obsessive-compulsive personality disorder

A. Characteristics
1. Preoccupation with order and rules
2. Perfectionism
3. Tendency to prescribe how others must do things
4. Inefficiency caused by constant worry over doing things correctly
5. Either anger or emotional constriction
6. Use of reaction formation, undoing, and displacement as primary defense mechanisms

B. Criteria for medical diagnosis (see the *DSM-III-R* diagnostic criteria for obsessive-compulsive personality disorder on pages 146 and 147)

C. Treatment
1. Behavioral therapies
2. Cognitive therapies
3. Leisure activities

(Text continues on page 147.)

Diagnostic criteria for personality disorders

The following chart presents the *DSM-III-R* diagnostic criteria for the personality disorders discussed in this chapter. The criteria refer to behaviors or traits characteristic of the person's recent (past year) and long-term functioning (generally since adolescence or early adulthood). These behaviors or traits cause subjective distress or significant impairment in social or occupational functioning. Behaviors or traits limited to episodes of illness are not considered when diagnosing a personality disorder.

Paranoid personality disorder
A. The person exhibits a pervasive and unwarranted tendency, beginning by early adulthood and present in various contexts, to interpret the actions of others as deliberately demeaning or threatening, as indicated by at least four of the following:
  1. Expects, without sufficient basis, to be exploited or harmed by others
  2. Questions, without justification, the loyalty or trustworthiness of friends or associates
  3. Reads hidden demeaning or threatening meanings into benign remarks or events (such as suspecting that a neighbor has put out the trash early to cause annoyance)
  4. Bears grudges or is unforgiving of insults or slights
  5. Is reluctant to confide in others because of unwarranted fear that the information will be used against him or her
  6. Is easily slighted and quick to react with anger or to counterattack
  7. Questions, without justification, fidelity of spouse or sexual partner
B. The disturbance does not occur exclusively during the course of schizophrenia or a delusional disorder

Schizoid personality disorder
A. The person exhibits a pervasive pattern of indifference to social relationships and a restricted range of emotional experience and expression, beginning by early adulthood and present in various contexts, as indicated by at least four of the following:
  1. Neither desires nor enjoys close relationships, including being part of a family
  2. Almost always chooses solitary activities
  3. Rarely, if ever, claims or appears to experience strong emotions, such as anger and joy
  4. Indicates little, if any, desire to have sexual experiences with another person (age being taken into account)
  5. Is indifferent to the praise and criticism of others
  6. Has no close friends or confidants (or only one) other than first-degree relatives
  7. Displays constricted affect (is aloof and cold; rarely reciprocates gestures or facial expressions, such as smiles or nods)
B. The disturbance does not occur exclusively during the course of schizophrenia or a delusional disorder

Schizotypal personality disorder
A. The person exhibits a pervasive pattern of deficits in interpersonal relatedness and peculiarities of ideation, appearance, and behavior, beginning by early adulthood and present in various contexts, as indicated by at least five of the following:
  1. Ideas of reference (excluding delusions of reference)

Diagnostic criteria for personality disorders *(continued)*

2. Excessive social anxiety (for example, extreme discomfort in social situations involving unfamiliar people)
3. Odd beliefs or magical thinking that influences behavior and is inconsistent with subcultural norms, such as superstitiousness, belief in clairvoyance, telepathy (in children and adolescents, bizarre fantasies or preoccupations)
4. Unusual perceptual experiences, such as illusions, sensing the presence of a force or person not actually present (for example, "I felt as if my dead mother were in the room with me")
5. Odd or eccentric behavior or appearance (is unkempt, displays unusual mannerisms, talks to self)
6. No close friends or confidants (or only one) other than first-degree relatives
7. Odd speech (without loosening of associations or incoherence), such as speech that is impoverished, digressive, vague, or inappropriately abstract
8. Inappropriate or constricted affect (is silly or aloof; rarely reciprocates gestures or facial expressions, such as smiles or nods)
9. Suspiciousness or paranoid ideation

B. The disturbance does not occur exclusively during the course of schizophrenia or a pervasive developmental disorder

Antisocial personality disorder

A. The person is age 18 or older

B. The person's history includes evidence of conduct disorder with onset before age 15, as indicated by three or more of the following:
1. Was often truant
2. Ran away from home overnight at least twice while living in parental or parental surrogate home (or once without returning)
3. Often initiated physical fights
4. Used a weapon in more than one fight
5. Forced someone into sexual activity
6. Was physically cruel to animals
7. Was physically cruel to other people
8. Deliberately destroyed others' property (other than by arson)
9. Deliberately engaged in arson
10. Often lied (other than to avoid physical or sexual abuse)
11. Has stolen without confrontation of a victim on more than one occasion (including forgery)
12. Has stolen with confrontation of a victim (such as mugging, purse-snatching, extortion, or armed robbery)

C. The person exhibits a pattern of irresponsible and antisocial behavior since the age of 15, as indicated by at least four of the following:
1. Is unable to sustain consistent work behavior, as indicated by any of the following (including similar behavior in academic settings if the person is a student):
   a. Significant unemployment for 6 months or more within 5 years when expected to work and work was available

(continued)

Diagnostic criteria for personality disorders *(continued)*

      b. Repeated absences from work unexplained by illness in self or family

      c. Abandonment of several jobs without realistic plans for others

  2. Fails to conform to social norms with respect to lawful behavior, as indicated by repeatedly performing antisocial acts that are grounds for arrest (whether arrested or not), such as destroying property, harassing others, stealing, or pursuing an illegal occupation

  3. Is irritable and aggressive, as indicated by repeated physical fights or assaults (not required by one's job or to defend someone or oneself), including spouse- or child-beating

  4. Repeatedly fails to honor financial obligations, as indicated by defaulting on debts or failing to provide child support for other dependents on a regular basis

  5. Fails to plan ahead, or is impulsive, as indicated by one or both of the following:

      a. Traveling from place to place without a prearranged job or clear goal for the period of travel or a clear idea about when the travel will terminate

      b. Lack of a fixed address for 1 month or more

  6. Has no regard for the truth, as indicated by repeated lying, use of aliases, or conning others for personal profit or pleasure

  7. Is reckless regarding personal safety or the safety of others, as indicated by driving while intoxicated or recurrent speeding

  8. Lacks ability to function as a responsible parent, as indicated by one or more of the following:

      a. Malnutrition of child

      b. Child's illness resulting from lack of minimal hygiene

      c. Failure to obtain medical care for a seriously ill child

      d. Child's dependence on neighbors or nonresident relatives for food or shelter

      e. Failure to arrange for a caregiver for young child when parent is away from home

      f. Repeated squandering, on personal items, of money required for household necessities

  9. Has never sustained a monogamous relationship for more than 1 year

  10. Lacks remorse (feels justified in having hurt, mistreated, or stolen from another)

D. Antisocial behavior does not occur exclusively during the course of schizophrenia or manic episodes

Borderline personality disorder

The person exhibits a pervasive pattern of instability of mood, interpersonal relationships, and self-image, beginning by early adulthood and present in various contexts, as indicated by at least five of the following:

  1. A pattern of unstable and intense interpersonal relationships characterized by alternating between extremes of overidealization and devaluation

  2. Impulsiveness in at least two areas that are potentially self-damaging, such as spending, sex, substance use, shoplifting, reckless driving, or binge eating (do not include suicidal or self-mutilating behavior covered in criterion 5)

  3. Affective instability: that is, marked shifts from baseline mood to depression, irritability, or anxiety, usually lasting a few hours and only rarely more than a few days

Diagnostic criteria for personality disorders *(continued)*

4. Inappropriate, intense anger or lack of control of anger, such as frequent displays of temper, constant anger, or recurrent physical fights
5. Recurrent suicidal threats, gestures, or behavior, or self-mutilating behavior
6. Marked and persistent identity disturbance manifested by uncertainty about at least two of the following: self-image, sexual orientation, long-term goals or career choice, type of friends desired, preferred values
7. Chronic feelings of emptiness or boredom
8. Frantic efforts to avoid real or imagined abandonment (do not include suicidal or self-mutilating behavior covered in criterion 5)

Histrionic personality disorder

The person exhibits a pervasive pattern of excessive emotionality and attention-seeking, beginning by early adulthood and present in various contexts, as indicated by at least four of the following:

1. Constantly seeks or demands reassurance, approval, or praise
2. Is inappropriately sexually seductive in appearance or behavior
3. Is overly concerned with physical attractiveness
4. Expresses emotion with inappropriate exaggeration (for example, embraces casual acquaintances with excessive ardor, sobs uncontrollably on minor sentimental occasions, has temper tantrums)
5. Is uncomfortable when not the center of attention
6. Displays rapidly shifting and shallow expression of emotions
7. Is self-centered, with actions being directed toward obtaining immediate satisfaction; has no tolerance for the frustration of delayed gratification
8. Has a style of speech that is excessively impressionistic and lacking in detail (for example, when asked to describe mother, can be no more specific than "She was a beautiful person")

Narcissistic personality disorder

The person exhibits a pervasive pattern of grandiosity (in fantasy or behavior), lack of empathy, and hypersensitivity to the evaluation of others, beginning by early adulthood and present in various contexts, as indicated by at least five of the following:

1. Reacts to criticism with feelings of rage, shame, or humiliation (even if not expressed)
2. Is interpersonally exploitative: takes advantage of others to achieve personal ends
3. Has a grandiose sense of self-importance (for example, exaggerates achievements and talents; expects to be noticed as "special" without appropriate achievement)
4. Believes that his or her problems are unique and can be understood only by other special people
5. Is preoccupied with fantasies of unlimited success, power, brilliance, beauty, or ideal love
6. Has a sense of entitlement: that is, unreasonable expectation of especially favorable treatment (for example, assumes that he or she does not have to wait in line when others must do so)
7. Requires constant attention and admiration; keeps fishing for compliments

(continued)

Diagnostic criteria for personality disorders *(continued)*

8. Lack of empathy: inability to recognize and experience how others feel (for instance, is annoyed and surprised when a seriously ill friend cancels a date)
9. Is preoccupied with feelings of envy

Avoidant personality disorder

The person exhibits a pervasive pattern of social discomfort, fear of negative evaluation, and timidity, beginning by early adulthood and present in a various contexts, as indicated by at least four of the following:

1. Is easily hurt by criticism or disapproval
2. Has no close friends or confidants (or only one) other than first-degree relatives
3. Is unwilling to get involved with people unless certain of being liked
4. Avoids social or occupational activities that involve significant interpersonal contact (for example, refuses a promotion that will increase social demands)
5. Is reticent in social situations because of a fear of saying something inappropriate or foolish, or of being unable to answer a question
6. Fears being embarrassed by blushing, crying, or showing signs of anxiety in front of other people
7. Exaggerates the potential difficulties, physical dangers, or risks involved in doing something ordinary but outside his or her usual routine (for example, may cancel social plans because he or she anticipates being exhausted by the effort of getting there)

Dependent personality disorder

The person exhibits a pervasive pattern of dependent and submissive behavior, beginning by early adulthood and present in various contexts, as indicated by at least five of the following:

1. Is unable to make everyday decisions without an excessive amount of advice or reassurance from others
2. Allows others to make most of his or her important decisions, such as where to live or which job to take
3. Agrees with people even when he or she believes they are wrong, for fear of being rejected
4. Has difficulty initiating projects or doing things independently
5. Volunteers to do things that are unpleasant or demeaning in order to be liked by others
6. Feels uncomfortable or helpless when alone or goes to great lengths to avoid being alone
7. Feels devastated or helpless when close relationships end
8. Is frequently preoccupied with fears of being abandoned
9. Is easily hurt by criticism or disapproval

Obsessive-compulsive personality disorder

The person exhibits a pervasive pattern of perfectionism and inflexibility, beginning by early adulthood and present in various contexts, as indicated by at least five of the following:

1. Perfectionism that interferes with task completion (such as inability to complete a project because one's overly strict standards are not met)
2. Preoccupation with details, rules, lists, order, organization, or schedules to the extent that the major point of the activity is lost

Diagnostic criteria for personality disorders *(continued)*

3. Unreasonable insistence that others submit to exactly his or her way of doing things, or unreasonable reluctance to allow others to do things because of the conviction that they will not do them correctly
4. Excessive devotion to work and productivity to the exclusion of leisure activities and friendships (not accounted for by obvious economic necessity)
5. Indecisiveness: decision making is either avoided, postponed, or protracted; for example, the person cannot get assignments done on time because of ruminating about priorities (do not include if indecisiveness is due to excessive need for advice or reassurance from others)
6. Overconscientiousness, scrupulousness, and inflexibility about matters of morality, ethics, or values (not accounted for by cultural or religious identification)
7. Restricted expression of affection
8. Lack of generosity in giving time, money, or gifts when no personal gain is likely to result
9. Inability to discard worn-out or worthless objects even when they have no sentimental value

Passive-aggressive personality disorder

The person exhibits a pervasive pattern of passive resistance to demands for adequate social and occupational performance, beginning by early adulthood and present in various contexts, as indicated by at least five of the following:

1. Procrastinates (postpones tasks that need to be done so that deadlines are not met)
2. Becomes sulky, irritable, or argumentative when asked to do something he or she does not want to do
3. Seems to work deliberately slowly or to do a bad job on tasks that he or she really does not want to do
4. Protests, without justification, that others make unreasonable demands on him or her
5. Avoids obligations by claiming to have "forgotten"
6. Believes that he or she is doing a much better job than others think he or she is doing
7. Resents useful suggestions from others concerning how he or she could be more productive
8. Obstructs the efforts of others by failing to do his or her share of the work
9. Unreasonably criticizes or scorns people in positions of authority

Source: *Diagnostic and Statistical Manual of Mental Disorders,* Third Edition-Revised. Washington, D.C.: American Psychiatric Association, 1987. Adapted with permission.

   D. Possible nursing diagnoses
      1. Sleep pattern disturbance related to preoccupation with obsessive-compulsive behaviors
      2. Anxiety related to the need for perfection
      3. Altered health maintenance related to difficulty in completing activities of daily living

E. General nursing interventions
1. Assist the client in becoming more flexible and in generating alternative solutions to life situations
2. Confront invalid assumptions so the client can reassess a situation and develop a new perspective

XIII. Passive-aggressive personality disorder

A. Characteristics
1. Passive hostility
2. Inefficiency (typified by tendencies to put off the completion of tasks and to forget commitments that the client has made)
3. Covert resentment of those who make legitimate demands on the client
4. Criticism of others
5. Steadfast refusal to alter behavior
6. Passive anger
7. Underlying depression
8. Use of passive aggression as a primary defense mechanism

B. Criteria for medical diagnosis (see the *DSM-III-R* diagnostic criteria for passive-aggressive personality disorder on page 147)

C. Treatment
1. Assertiveness training
2. Relaxation exercises

D. Possible nursing diagnoses
1. Ineffective individual coping related to denial of hostile feelings
2. Noncompliance with the treatment plan related to lack of insight about the disorder
3. Ineffective family coping related to secondary gains

E. General nursing interventions
1. Foster the client's assertiveness
2. Teach the client appropriate ways to express underlying feelings

Clinical situation

Kay, age 29, is admitted to your psychiatric unit for treatment and evaluation after an episode of self-mutilation. She inflicted the injury after her boyfriend of 1 week cancelled a date with her because he had to work late. Kay now has been on the unit for about 48 hours. During this time, she has had several angry outbursts about the physicians and nurses not being able to meet with her on demand. She vacillates between saying she wants to turn her life around and saying that she is a horrible person who should be allowed to die. Kay's diagnosis on admission is borderline personality disorder.

As Kay's primary nurse, you have contracted to spend two 30-minute blocks of time with her on an individual basis each day. However, Kay says she needs more time with you, and she manages to get you to spend up to 4 hours per shift with her by telling you that you are the only one she can trust, the only one who "really cares" about her.

Kay spends much of her time on the phone, complaining to friends about how badly she is being treated in the hospital. She also tries several times to contact her new boyfriend, and when her attempts prove unsuccessful, she uses profane language and throws a chair. When not on the phone, Kay hangs around the nurses' station, demanding to be seen, or sits in the day room with a male client. Staff members have observed them holding hands, rubbing each other's backs, and engaging in prolonged kissing. Kay is now demanding off-unit privileges because remaining on the unit is "boring as hell."

Assessment (nursing behaviors and rationales)

1. Assess Kay's potential for further self-mutilation and for suicide. *Ensuring the client's safety is the nurse's top priority when caring for a client with borderline personality disorder. Self-mutilation is a primary characteristic of this disorder, and suicide attempts are commonplace. Knowing the client's state of mind about self-destruction provides data for planning appropriate care.*

2. Assess Kay's ability to control her impulses. *The client's potential for acting-out behavior places her and others at risk for injury.*

3. Assess Kay's level of ego functioning. *This assessment provides information about the client's strengths and weaknesses.*

4. Assess the effect that Kay is having on staff and other clients. *Power struggles are inevitable when caring for a client with borderline personality disorder. Unless staff members remain clear on what needs to be addressed—and by whom, how, and when—the client may succeed in causing dissension among the staff, which would be detrimental to all parties.*

Nursing diagnoses

- High risk for violence related to poor impulse control
- Ineffective individual coping related to immature ego structure
- Noncompliance with the treatment plan related to power struggles between the client and authority figures
- Impaired social interaction related to underlying fear of abandonment

Planning and goals

- Kay will not harm herself or others while hospitalized.
- Kay will practice age-appropriate coping skills.
- Kay will follow a written contract for compliance with treatment protocols.

Implementation (nursing behaviors and rationales)

1. Teach Kay problem-solving skills she can use to interrupt acting-out behaviors when feeling abandoned, lonely, afraid, or angry. *This will help the client learn that her responses to situations are stimulated by underlying negative feelings that are related to external events. Such insight will probably empower the client to remain in control.*

2. Provide Kay with a consistent environment by strictly adhering to the agreed-upon treatment plan and by using written contracts that you mutually review each day. *Such consistency creates a "holding" environment in which the client* *can feel safe. Written contracts greatly reduce ambiguities and game playing. Daily review of the contracts promotes a consistent treatment approach, permits each party to clarify any misunderstandings, and allows for timely updating as needed.*

3. Hold daily staff conferences to address all problems that result from Kay's maladaptive behaviors. *Daily sessions will severely curtail the client's ability to cause dissension among staff members and will provide the staff with a vehicle for airing concerns relating to the client's care.*

4. Use rational authority when enforcing limits that are defined by unit policy or written contract. *Consistent, dispassionate limit setting will greatly enhance the client's feelings of security, eventually eliminate power struggles, and ultimately increase the client's ability to predict future events based on consistent past experiences. Furthermore, rational authority helps staff members avoid personalizing their actions or feeling responsible either for the client's behaviors or for the resulting consequences.*

5. Develop specific schedules for contracts between Kay and staff members. *Like other clients with borderline personality disorder, the client in this clinical situation fears abandonment. She acts out and behaves inappropriately to compel others to be in her proximity. If she knows when to expect contact with staff, she may better tolerate the times when she must be alone.*

6. Specify the rules that Kay must follow when relating to other clients and the consequences that she must face if she ignores the rules. *Staff members have an obligation to protect other clients from this client's seductive ploys. Because of the nature of her illness, she will be a master at exploiting others to meet her needs. They, in turn, are at risk for emotional or physical harm.*

Evaluation

- Kay does not harm herself or others while hospitalized.
- Kay learns to delay gratification by identifying her needs and by selecting rational, age-appropriate ways to meet these needs.
- Kay practices relaxation techniques when she becomes aware of feeling anxious.
- Kay participates in a support group for individuals with borderline personality disorder.
- Kay sets realistic daily goals.

16 Schizophrenia

I. Overview

A. Schizophrenia is the most commonly diagnosed thought disorder

B. It is characterized by severe, prolonged disturbances of affect; withdrawal from reality; regressive behavior; poor communications; and impaired interpersonal relationships (see the *DSM-III-R* diagnostic criteria for schizophrenia on pages 155 and 156)

C. Onset begins with a notable impairment in some areas of daily functioning, such as work, social relationships, or self-care

D. The person's premorbid personality is usually described as suspicious, introverted, withdrawn, eccentric, and impulsive

E. The person reports feeling "strange," is confused about the origin of the impairment, and develops a sense of being separate and different from others

F. Life expectancy among those with schizophrenia is shortened because of an increased likelihood of suicide

G. The disorder usually begins during adolescence or early adulthood but can develop in middle or late adulthood

II. Theoretical perspectives

A. Biological theories

    1. Genetic theory

        a. About 10% of first-degree relatives (immediate family members, such as mother and father, brothers and sisters, sons and daughters) are diagnosed with schizophrenia at some point during their lives

        b. Studies of twins point to both genetic and environmental factors; for instance, concordance rates (those in which both twins either show or do not show the schizophrenic trait) consistently are higher for monozygotic twins than for dizygotic twins

    2. Biochemical theory

        a. Dopamine causes overactive neuronal activity; drugs that decrease dopamine activity decrease psychotic symptoms

        b. Norepinephrine is highly concentrated in the hypothalamus, thalamus, limbic system, and cerebellum of a schizophrenic client

    B. Psychological theory

        1. A person with schizophrenia has an information-processing deficit; that is, an inability to control or discriminate the information being received

        2. A person with schizophrenia has an impaired ability to make comparisons among stimuli and to organize them sequentially or logically

    C. Family theory

        1. The disorder results from communication problems within families that have genetic vulnerability to schizophrenia

        2. Highly charged emotional family life and disturbed communications within families contribute to schizophrenia

    D. Psychoanalytic theory

        1. The person's ego cannot cope with pressure from the id and reality because of a disrupted mother-child relationship

        2. The child receives mixed and confused communication from the mother and significant others before developing an ability to clarify meaning

        3. The resulting stress and anxiety cause continued disintegration of the ego, leading to thought disturbances

    E. Biosocioenvironmental theory

        1. The interaction between the person and the environment influences the development of the disorder

        2. The occurrence of schizophrenia is related to the environment and to one's inner strength and vulnerability to stress

III. Signs and symptoms

    A. Language and communications disturbances

        1. A person with schizophrenia cannot maintain a consistent, logical train of thought

        2. Reasoning usually follows the person's own unfathomable private rules

        3. The person shows poverty of speech and may begin to form neologisms in severe stages of the disorder

    B. Thought disturbances

        1. Delusions, particularly those about the person's thoughts being read by others, are characteristic

        2. Ideas of reference and persecution delusions are intense

    C. Perceptual disturbances

        1. Auditory hallucinations are the most common type

        2. Voices communicate directly with the person, criticizing the person's thoughts and behavior

D. Affect disturbances

    1. The demonstrable emotion is labile or flat and commonly is inappropriate

    2. The person will typically complain of losing "normal feelings"

E. Motor behavior disturbances

    1. The person may be in a state of constant, wildly bizarre, and aggressive activity that can lead to profound exhaustion

    2. Conversely, the motor disturbance can produce a marked decrease in activity, leading to a virtual cessation of spontaneous movement (catatonia)

F. Self-identity disturbances

    1. The person loses a sense of self-identity

    2. The person believes that mysterious forces are changing the person's core being; a sense of nothingness develops

IV. Behavioral types of schizophrenia

A. Paranoid type

    1. Primary characteristics include persecutory delusions and hallucinations

    2. Communications break down because of the person's extreme suspicion, which leads to reduced levels of functioning and withdrawn behavior

B. Catatonic type

    1. The primary characteristic is either increased motor excitement or stuporous, rigid, posturing behavior

    2. The extreme withdrawal helps the person control fear and anxiety

C. Disorganized type

    1. Primary characteristics include incoherent speech, unsystematized delusions, and inappropriate, silly affect

    2. The disturbance produces marked functional impairment with a poor outlook for remission

D. Undifferentiated type

    1. Primary characteristics include grossly disorganized, incoherent behavior; hallucinations; and prominent delusions

    2. The person's functioning level is severely impaired

E. Residual type

    1. The primary characteristic is a lack of schizophrenic symptoms, although the person has had a previous schizophrenic episode

    2. Functioning level is moderate, but the person rarely can keep a job

V. Treatment

A. Psychosocial therapy

    1. This form of therapy initially focuses on the client's physical safety

    2. Once the client's safety has been established, health care personnel form a therapeutic alliance with the client to understand the client's behavior and to support the client in abandoning maladaptive behaviors for more acceptable ones

    3. Therapists then design a treatment plan to raise the client's functioning level and to educate the family on how to respond to the client's behavior

    4. A team approach — one that involves a psychiatrist or psychologist, a nurse, and a social worker — is used to carry out the treatment plan

B. Drug therapy

    1. Phenothiazine and neuroleptic agents have been remarkably effective in restoring the client's functioning level so that the client can return to society

    2. Drug treatment may consist of low-potency or high-potency drugs, depending on the treatment strategies adopted to relieve psychotic symptoms

    3. Adjunctive drugs, such as anticholinergic agents, propranolol, or diphenhydramine, may be used to control adverse effects

C. Combination therapy

    1. Although drug treatment can help normalize a client's behavior, it has marginal effect on improving the client's social skills or overall quality of life

    2. Long-term treatment requires building a stable psychological foundation and helping the client accept responsibility for self-care, the development of social relationships, and vocational satisfaction

VI. Possible nursing diagnoses

A. Altered thought processes related to inability to trust, an underdeveloped ego, and biochemical imbalances

B. Ineffective individual coping related to low self-esteem

C. Social isolation related to lack of trust and delusional thinking

D. Self-care deficit related to regression to an earlier developmental level

E. Sensory-perceptual alterations related to hallucinations

F. Impaired verbal communication related to withdrawn behavior

G. High risk for violence directed at others related to suspiciousness

H. Noncompliance with the treatment plan related to suspiciousness and lack of insight

Diagnostic criteria for schizophrenia

The following chart presents the *DSM-III-R* diagnostic criteria for schizophrenia.

A. The person exhibits characteristic psychotic symptoms in the active phase (1, 2, or 3 below) for at least 1 week (unless the symptoms are successfully treated)
  1. At least two of the following:
    a. Delusions
    b. Prominent hallucinations (throughout the day for several days or several times a week for several weeks, each hallucinatory experience not being limited to a few brief moments)
    c. Incoherence or marked loosening of associations
    d. Catatonic behavior
    e. Flat or grossly inappropriate affect
  2. Bizarre delusions (that is, involving a phenomenon that the person's culture would regard as totally implausible, such as thought broadcasting or being controlled by a dead person)
  3. Prominent hallucinations (as defined in 1b above) of a voice with content having no apparent relation to depression or elation, or a voice keeping up a running commentary on the person's behavior or thoughts, or two or more voices conversing with each other

B. During the course of the disturbance, functioning in such areas as work, social relations, and self-care is markedly below the highest level achieved before onset of the disturbance (or, when the onset is in childhood or adolescence, failure to achieve expected level of social development)

C. Schizoaffective disorder and mood disorder with psychotic features have been ruled out (that is, if a major depressive or manic syndrome has ever been present during an active phase of the disturbance, the total duration of all episodes of a mood syndrome has been brief relative to the total duration of the active and residual phases of the disturbance)

D. The person exhibits continuous signs of the disturbance for at least 6 months
  1. The 6-month period must include an active phase of at least 1 week (or less, if symptoms have been successfully treated)
  2. The active phase must include psychotic symptoms characteristic of schizophrenia (symptoms in criterion A above), with or without a prodromal or residual phase, as defined below
    a. Prodromal phase: clear deterioration in functioning before the active phase of the disturbance that is not due to a disturbance in mood or to a psychoactive substance use disorder and that involves at least two of the symptoms listed below
    b. Residual phase: following the active phase of the disturbance, persistence of at least two of the symptoms noted below, these not being due to a disturbance in mood or to a psychoactive substance use disorder
    c. Prodromal or residual symptoms:
      (1) Marked social isolation or withdrawal
      (2) Marked impairment in role functioning as wage-earner, student, or homemaker
      (3) Markedly peculiar behavior (such as collecting garbage, talking to oneself in public, hoarding food)

(continued)

Diagnostic criteria for schizophrenia *(continued)*

    (4) Marked impairment in personal hygiene and grooming

    (5) Blunted or inappropriate affect

    (6) Digressive, vague, overelaborate, or circumstantial speech, or poverty of speech, or poverty of content of speech

    (7) Odd beliefs or magical thinking that influences behavior and is inconsistent with cultural norms (superstitiousness, belief in clairvoyance or telepathy, overvalued ideas, ideas of reference)

    (8) Unusual perceptual experiences (recurrent illusions, sensing the presence of a force or person not actually present)

    (9) Marked lack of initiative, interests, or energy

    Examples: 6 months of prodromal symptoms with 1 week of symptoms from A; no prodromal symptoms with 6 months of symptoms from A; no prodromal symptoms with 1 week of symptoms from A and 6 months of residual symptoms

E. It cannot be established that an organic factor initiated and maintained the disturbance

F. If there is a history of autistic disorder, the additional diagnosis of schizophrenia is made only if prominent delusions or hallucinations are also present

Source: *Diagnostic and Statistical Manual of Mental Disorders,* Third Edition-Revised. Washington, D.C.: American Psychiatric Association, 1987. Adapted with permission.

VII. General nursing interventions

A. Safety

    1. Remove any unsafe objects from the client's environment

    2. Reassure the client that the environment is safe by explaining procedures used to provide protection

    3. Monitor the client for increased psychomotor activity, intensity of affect, and verbalization or carrying out of delusional thinking

B. Environment

    1. Keep the client oriented to reality

    2. Minimize environmental stimuli

    3. Reassure other clients that their behavior did not provoke the client's threats

    4. Communicate in clear, direct, and concise statements

C. Self-esteem

    1. Assist the client with grooming, if needed

    2. Allow the client to make decisions when appropriate

    3. Acknowledge the client's abilities and skills, and use them to reinforce teaching

D. Social activities

    1. Assist the client in identifying life-style patterns that can be used to build better social relationships

2. Help the client evaluate the effectiveness of communication skills and social interactions

3. Give positive reinforcement when the client voluntarily interacts with others

4. Encourage the client to participate in group activities

E. Ego development

1. Validate client perceptions that are accurate, and correct misperceptions

2. Spend time with the client even when the client cannot respond coherently

3. Convey acceptance of the client while attempting to correct unacceptable behavior

4. Give praise and encouragement when the client chooses socially acceptable methods of managing anger and aggression

F. Homeostasis

1. Monitor the client's vital signs

2. Provide periods for adequate sleep

3. Provide a nutritious diet

4. Control hyperactive psychomotor activity

Clinical situation

John Ellis, age 36, is admitted to your psychiatric unit for the third time with a diagnosis of schizophrenia. The day before, he had been arrested for intimately touching a woman he didn't know, without her consent. Then, while in jail awaiting arraignment, he burned himself with matches he had hidden. The injury required treatment at the local hospital's emergency department, where he reportedly hit his father, who had come to see him.

Now, on arrival at the psychiatric facility, John is in handcuffs, yelling repeatedly. He appears restless, agitated, demanding, suspicious, and paranoid, and he exhibits looseness of association. John admits to auditory hallucinations and seems out of contact with reality. For the past year, according to his medical records, he has been taking Thorazine 100 mg b.i.d., Stelazine 20 mg b.i.d., and Cogentin 1 mg in the morning.

Assessment (nursing behaviors and rationales)

1. Assess John's potential for violence against others or self. *If the client exhibits suicidal tendencies or overt hostile and aggressive behaviors, the nurse and other staff members will need to take precautions to protect the client and others from harm.*

2. Assess John's personal hygiene, sleep pattern, and motor activity level. *This assessment will provide data that the nurse can use to determine the amount of nursing assistance that the client requires.*

3. Assess John's coping pattern, social support, financial status, educational level, and patterns of interactions with others. *This assessment will provide information about perceived and actual coping ability, developmental level, and problem-solving ability. It also will help determine the availability of family and friends to assist in the client's recovery.*

4. Assess the type of hallucinations and delusions that John is experiencing. *Information obtained from this assessment will reveal the extent of the client's disorganized thinking.*

5. Conduct a thorough physical examination. *A physical examination will provide data about possible organic causes for behavior.*

Nursing diagnoses

• Altered thought processes related to impaired judgment
• Sensory-perceptual alteration related to auditory hallucinations
• Social isolation related to distrust of others
• High risk for self-directed violence related to lack of trust and delusional thinking
• Self-care deficit related to withdrawn behavior and inattention to personal grooming

Planning and goals

• John will remain oriented to reality by controlling his behavior.
• John will maintain a satisfactory balance of nutritious diet, adequate sleep, and proper exercise.
• John will not harm others or himself.
• John will participate in the therapeutic environment.

Implementation *(nursing behaviors and rationales)*

1. Focus the client on reality. Do not reinforce delusional thinking, but acknowledge its presence. *Acknowledging delusional thinking and searching for what might have triggered it are the first steps toward defusing it.*

2. Provide for uninterrupted sleep as much as possible. *With adequate sleep, the client will experience less physical and psychological stress and will exhibit fewer bizarre behaviors.*

3. Establish a pattern of therapeutic communication. *Effective communication can facilitate the development of the therapeutic nurse-client relationship and can help the client in working through the problem-solving process.*

4. Monitor vital signs and provide for John's physical needs. *Systematic monitoring will alert the nurse to a change in the client's functional status and the need for prompt intervention.*

5. Do not argue with John about his delusions or hallucinations. *Altered perceptions frighten the client and indicate loss of control. Because of lack of insight, this client views his delusions and hallucinations as reality. Arguing only leads to defensiveness.*

6. Establish a daily routine for John. *The client's ability to adapt is severely impaired. A well-maintained routine will be less threatening to him.*

7. Monitor the frequency of hallucinations and the intensity of delusions. *Command hallucinations or delusions may precede bizarre, destructive, or suicidal behavior.*

8. Teach John basic social skills, such as conversation. *The client may never have learned how to carry on a social conversation, such as discussing the weather or a sporting event. Developing basic social skills can help build the* *client's self-confidence, enhance self-esteem, and reduce anxiety, all of which contribute to social acceptance.*

9. Direct John toward activities that will decrease the likelihood of his acting on hallucinatory or delusional misinterpretations. *Redirecting the client's energies to more acceptable activities will help reduce the likelihood of inappropriate behavior.*

10. Provide opportunities for John to accept responsibility and make decisions. *The client must gain a sense of independence before he can be discharged. Accepting responsibility for behavior and participating in decision making will enhance the client's self-confidence and promote his sense of independence.*

11. Teach John and family members about John's condition. Review the importance of taking medications as prescribed, and discuss their adverse effects. *To ensure proper care at home and to promote compliance with treatment, the client and his family must have accurate information about his illness, treatment, and effects of medications.*

Evaluation
- John follows an adequate diet and maintains a proper balance of sleep and exercise.
- John demonstrates increased self-esteem.
- John becomes independent in self-care.
- John engages in community social activities.
- John accurately repeats the instructions for taking his medication and can recite their adverse effects.

17 Somatoform disorders

I. Overview

    A. Somatoform disorders are a group of psychological conditions characterized by complaints of physical symptoms or illness for which no organic or physiologic cause exists

    B. The client typically has a lengthy history of diagnostic workups with negative physical findings, leading the health care professional to suspect a psychological cause for the physical symptoms

    C. The client does not have conscious control of the symptoms, which feel real to the client

    D. The psychological origin of these disorders is thought to be repressed anxiety
        1. The primary gain is that the symptoms allow the client to avoid the awareness of an internal conflict or need
        2. The symptoms represent, and partially solve, an underlying conflict

    E. Symptom formation and apparent disability are reinforced by a secondary gain, in which the person avoids a particularly unpleasant action and elicits support from others

    F. Clients with somatoform disorders are commonly seen first by physicians for treatment of perceived medical symptoms

    G. The differentiating diagnostic factor is the absence of any physiologic origin for the symptoms

II. Theoretical perspectives

    A. Psychoanalytic theory
        1. Freud postulated that successful psychological development depended on satisfying specific physical functions, such as eating
        2. Physical symptoms in somatoform disorders signal intrapsychic conflict from failure to meet earlier developmental needs

    B. Holistic theory
        1. Mental and physiologic processes are directly linked
        2. Any illness is both physical and psychological, each affecting the other

C. Stress theory

    1. Stress, even unconscious stress, can cause psychophysiologic disorders

    2. Hans Selye's generalized adaptation syndrome proposed three levels of response to stress

        a. Alarm reaction: the body is put into a "fight or flight" stance

        b. Stage of resistance: the body reduces its optimum level of function

        c. Stage of exhaustion: the body's adaptive ability fails, and death becomes imminent

III. Body dysmorphic disorder

    A. Characteristics

        1. Preoccupation with an imaginary defect in one's physical appearance, even though the person appears normal to others

        2. Complaints of facial flaws (or flaws in other parts of the body)

        3. Slight physical abnormality, but the person's preoccupation with it is out of proportion to the magnitude of the abnormality

        4. Primary incidence in young people

        5. Tendency to seek unnecessary surgery to correct the imaginary defect or minor flaw

        6. Possible impairment of social skills and work performance resulting from the client's desire to hide the perceived flaw

    B. Criteria for medical diagnosis (see the *DSM-III-R* diagnostic criteria for body dysmorphic disorder on page 165)

    C. Treatment

        1. Cognitive or other forms of psychotherapy

        2. Psychotropic medication to relieve associated depression and anxiety

    D. Possible nursing diagnoses

        1. Anxiety related to perceived physical flaw

        2. Ineffective individual coping related to alarm from perceiving a gross deformity

        3. High risk for injury related to unnecessary surgery

        4. Body image disturbance related to perceived disfigurement

    E. General nursing interventions

        1. Listen to the client's complaints empathetically

        2. Support the client's attempts to acknowledge that the existence or extent of the defect may be exaggerated

        3. Accompany the client to activities that are too uncomfortable for the client to attend alone

        4. Administer prescribed medications, and teach the client about their adverse effects

IV. Conversion disorder

A. Characteristics

1. Alteration or loss of functioning of a body part that is not related to any physical abnormalities

2. Symptoms not under the client's conscious control

   a. May be either disturbing to the client or not acknowledged at all (la belle indifference)

   b. Classically mimic neurologic problems, such as paralysis, blindness, aphonia, and other sensory disturbances

   c. May involve gastrointestinal or other systems

   d. Appear to express a conflict or an unmet need; primary and secondary gains are in operation

   e. Can be a single symptom of a presenting illness that may migrate or vary in subsequent episodes

   f. Can be multiple symptoms that severely constrict the client's ability to function, resulting in actual physical impairment from disuse of the body part

B. Criteria for medical diagnosis (see the *DSM-III-R* diagnostic criteria for conversion disorder on page 165)

C. Treatment

1. Thorough physical workup for each new presenting symptom

2. Psychotherapy to enable the client to acknowledge and resolve unconscious conflict

3. Physical rehabilitation for muscle atrophy, if indicated

4. Medication to relieve associated anxiety and depression

D. Possible nursing diagnoses

1. Ineffective individual coping related to feelings of inadequacy

2. Ineffective family coping (disabling) related to poor family relations

3. High risk for disuse syndrome related to loss of function of body part

4. Altered role performance related to physical conversion symptom

5. Hopelessness related to inability to resolve internal conflict

E. General nursing interventions

1. Allow the client to express feelings; listen empathetically and nonjudgmentally

2. Monitor and report any new conversion symptoms

3. Encourage self-care whenever possible to reduce secondary gains and dependence

4. Provide a safe environment for the client's particular impairment

5. Monitor for suicide potential

6. Support the family as they attempt to provide encouragement without providing secondary gain

V. Hypochondriasis

A. Characteristics

1. Morbid preoccupation with a fear or belief that one has a serious disease based on a personal interpretation of physical health
2. No physical evidence of serious disease
3. Unwavering conviction of illness; the client is neither delusional nor preoccupied with bodily functions
4. Anxiety, depression, and compulsive behavior
5. Avoidance of responsibility
6. Desire for attention
7. Manipulation of others

B. Criteria for medical diagnosis (see the *DSM-III-R* diagnostic criteria for hypochondriasis on page 165)

C. Treatment

1. Thorough physical examination and workup for each new conversion episode or complaint
2. Medication to reduce associated anxiety and depression
3. Psychotherapy, with the frequency of sessions related to the client's level of anxiety
4. Relaxation techniques

D. Possible nursing diagnoses

1. Anxiety related to ineffective coping ability
2. Altered health maintenance related to preoccupation with body functions
3. Ineffective individual coping related to denial of emotional problems
4. High risk for disuse syndrome from loss of function of a body part
5. Ineffective denial related to physical status
6. Knowledge deficit related to the illness

E. General nursing interventions

1. Allow the client to express concerns about physical symptoms; assume a nonjudgmental attitude
2. Offer the client health teaching about the illness, when appropriate
3. Teach and demonstrate relaxation techniques and other coping skills
4. Monitor and report any new conversion signs or symptoms
5. Monitor for suicide potential

VI. Somatization disorder

A. Characteristics

1. Many physical complaints or an ongoing conviction of serious illness occurring over many years
2. Dramatic but often vague communication of somatic complaints

3. Lack of organic or physiologic cause for symptoms
4. Possible appearance of other psychiatric diagnoses, such as anxiety and depression

B. Criteria for medical diagnosis (see the *DSM-III-R* diagnostic criteria for somatization disorder on pages 165 to 167)

C. Treatment
1. Thorough physical workup for each symptom
2. Genuine understanding by the health care professional that, although no physical cause may be evident, the client's distress and impairment are real and not consciously caused or controlled
3. Antidepressants and antianxiety medications, if prescribed
4. Psychotherapy to assist the client in dealing with unconscious conflicts and anxiety

D. Possible nursing diagnoses
1. Noncompliance with treatment related to pleasure gained from being sick
2. Ineffective individual coping related to use of physical illness as coping mechanism
3. Knowledge deficit related to inadequate understanding of the disorder
4. Self-esteem disturbance related to unsatisfactory interpersonal relationships

E. General nursing interventions
1. Monitor and report any new signs or symptoms
2. Listen objectively to the client, neither encouraging nor discouraging the expression of the client's symptoms
3. Discuss with the client a possible connection between emotions and physical symptoms
4. Protect the client's right to treatment and respect
5. Discuss the client's expectations about being in the hospital
6. Involve the client in planning care, setting goals, and selecting interventions

VII. Somatoform pain disorder

A. Characteristics
1. Preoccupation with pain without any diagnostic finding to account for the pain or its intensity
2. Pain that does not follow anatomical nervous system distribution (although the pain does feel real to the person and is not consciously being faked)

Diagnostic criteria for somatoform disorders

The following chart presents the *DSM-III-R* diagnostic criteria for the somatoform disorders discussed in this chapter.

Body dysmorphic disorder
A. The person has a preoccupation with some imagined defect in appearance, despite appearing normal to others; or, if a slight physical abnormality does exist, the person's concern is grossly excessive
B. The person has a nondelusional belief in the defect
C. The belief is unrelated to anorexia nervosa or transsexualism

Conversion disorder
A. The person experiences a loss of or alteration in physical functioning suggesting a physical disorder
B. Psychological factors are judged to be etiologically related to the symptom because of a temporal relationship between a psychosocial stressor that is apparently related to a psychological conflict or need and initiation or exacerbation of the symptom
C. The person is not conscious of intentionally producing the symptom
D. The symptom is not a culturally sanctioned response pattern and cannot, after appropriate investigation, be explained by a known physical disorder
E. The symptom is not limited to pain or to a disturbance in sexual functioning

Hypochondriasis
A. The person has a preoccupation with the fear of having, or the belief that he or she has, a serious disease, based on the person's interpretation of physical signs or sensations as evidence of physical illness
B. Appropriate physical evaluation does not support the diagnosis of any physical disorder that can account for the physical signs or sensations or the person's unwarranted interpretation of them, and the symptoms in criterion A are not just symptoms of panic attacks
C. The fear or belief persists despite medical reassurance
D. Duration of the disturbance is at least 6 months
E. The belief in criterion A is not of delusional intensity, as in delusional disorder, somatic type (that is, the person can acknowledge the possibility that his or her fear or belief is unfounded)

Somatization disorder
A. The person has a history of many physical complaints or a belief that he or she is sickly, beginning before age 30 and persisting for several years
B. Either of the following applies:
    1. No organic pathology or pathophysiologic mechanism (a physical disorder or the effects of injury, medication, drugs, or alcohol) accounts for the symptoms
    2. When related organic pathology does exist, the person's complaint or resulting social or occupational impairment grossly exceeds what would be expected from the physical findings

(continued)

Diagnostic criteria for somatoform disorders *(continued)*

C. Symptoms do not occur only during a panic attack
D. Symptoms are severe enough for the person to self-medicate (other than with nonprescription drugs), consult a physician, or change life-style
E. The person exhibits at least 13 of the following symptoms
   Gastrointestinal symptoms
   1. Vomiting (other than during pregnancy)
   2. Abdominal pain (other than when menstruating)
   3. Nausea (other than motion sickness)
   4. Bloating (flatulence)
   5. Diarrhea
   6. Intolerance of (gets sick from) several different foods
   Pain
   7. Extremities
   8. Back
   9. Joint
   10. On urination
   11. Other pain (excluding headaches)
   Cardiopulmonary symptoms
   12. Shortness of breath when not exerting oneself
   13. Palpitations
   14. Chest pain
   15. Dizziness
   Conversion or pseudoneurologic symptoms
   16. Amnesia
   17. Difficulty swallowing
   18. Loss of voice
   19. Deafness
   20. Double vision
   21. Blurred vision
   22. Blindness
   23. Fainting or loss of consciousness
   24. Seizures
   25. Difficulty walking
   26. Paralysis or muscle weakness
   27. Urine retention or difficulty urinating
   Sexual symptoms (for most of the person's life after having opportunities for sexual activity)
   28. Burning sensation in sexual organs or rectum (other than during intercourse)
   29. Sexual indifference
   30. Pain during intercourse
   31. Impotence
   Female reproductive symptoms (judged by the person to occur more frequently or severely than in most women)
   32. Painful menstruation
   33. Irregular menstrual periods

Diagnostic criteria for somatoform disorders *(continued)*

34. Excessive menstrual bleeding

35. Vomiting during the entire pregnancy

Note: Symptoms 1, 7, 12, 16, 17, 28, and 32 may be used to screen for the disorder. The presence of two or more of these symptoms suggests a high likelihood of the disorder.

Somatoform pain disorder

A. The person has a preoccupation with pain for at least 6 months

B. Either of the following applies

1. Appropriate evaluation uncovers no organic pathology or pathophysiologic mechanism (such as a physical disorder or the effects of injury) to account for the pain
2. When related organic pathology does exist, the complaint of pain or resulting social or occupational impairment grossly exceeds what would be expected from the physical findings

Source: *Diagnostic and Statistical Manual of Mental Disorders,* Third Edition-Revised. Washington, D.C.: American Psychiatric Association, 1987. Adapted with permission.

---

   3. Long history of physical complaints, consultations with numerous physicians, drug or alcohol abuse, and marked impairment of lifestyle

   4. Clear connection between a psychological stressor and onset of symptoms

   5. Possible secondary gain as a motivating factor in developing symptoms

B. Criteria for medical diagnosis (see the *DSM-III-R* diagnostic criteria for somatoform pain disorder in the chart above)

C. Treatment: Individual psychotherapy (most common approach in the absence of a definitive treatment for this condition)

D. Possible nursing diagnoses

   1. Anxiety related to severe pain

   2. Ineffective individual coping related to inability to deal with pain

   3. Impaired social interaction related to constant complaints of pain

   4. Altered role performance related to continual search for medical attention

E. General nursing interventions

   1. Monitor and report any new signs or symptoms

   2. Teach and reinforce relaxation techniques

   3. Acknowledge that the client is actually experiencing pain and distress while encouraging the client to explore feelings

   4. Reduce the opportunity for secondary gain by encouraging the client to perform as much self-care as possible

Clinical situation

Mr. Cruz, age 44, is admitted to the psychiatric ward of the Veterans' Administration Medical Center with a diagnosis of somatoform pain disorder. He has severe and debilitating pain in his back, radiating to his right leg, causing him to drag it.

The pain and paralysis have become increasingly severe over the last few months. Mr. Cruz reported that his first experience with this intense pain and resulting disability occurred while he was on leave from a tour of duty in Vietnam. He has been going to a medical clinic for several years, having many tests and examinations, with no definitive diagnoses.

He had two back surgeries, many other medical treatments, and numerous prescriptions for narcotic analgesics because of the pain. Mrs. Cruz revealed that her husband is now taking many more "pain pills" each day than were prescribed and that she is afraid he is becoming addicted to them. Comments by the referring emergency department staff indicated that they feel there is no organic cause for Mr. Cruz's pain and paralysis.

Mr. Cruz is painfully thin, with dark circles under his eyes and a perpetually sad expression. He speaks softly and is extremely cooperative. His gait is more of a drag than a walk; he pulls himself along by holding onto furniture or handrails. He complains of insomnia, decreased appetite, disinterest in sexual relations, a feeling of inadequacy as a parent and provider, and severe pain unrelieved by his prescription medications. He appears to lack insight into any possible psychological basis for his problem and, in fact, was quite upset by the repeated comments of emergency department staff that it was "all in his head."

Assessment (nursing behaviors and rationales)

1. Perform a physical assessment. *A physical assessment establishes baseline data and helps determine if additional testing is indicated.*

2. Perform a psychosocial and cultural assessment. *A psychosocial and cultural assessment provides information that the nurse can use to develop an individualized plan of care.*

3. Assess Mr. Cruz's perceptions of the problem. *This allows the client to describe, in his own words, the pain he is feeling and its possible cause. The client may minimize or exaggerate the physical problem.*

Nursing diagnoses

• Post-trauma response related to experiences in Vietnam
• Body image disturbance related to the inability to walk
• High risk for injury related to overuse of prescription pain relief medications

Planning and goals

• Mr. Cruz will feel less pain by the end of his hospitalization.
• Mr. Cruz will participate in a physical rehabilitation program to help regain the use of his right leg.
• Mr. Cruz will participate in ongoing psychotherapy to assist in his difficulties with role performance.

Implementation (nursing behaviors and rationales)

1. Redirect Mr. Cruz's attention away from himself by contracting to engage in diversional activities. *The client's preoccupation with his pain and health status must be disrupted before he can begin to understand how his condition developed.*

2. Encourage Mr. Cruz to express his feelings about his work and family. *The client needs to develop an awareness of his emotional life and to resolve those feelings that may cause him physical pain.*

3. Provide emotional support. *The client probably feels alone and uncared for. Emotional support from the nurse may increase his sense of belonging and self-worth.*

4. Teach techniques that will reduce Mr. Cruz's anxiety. *A client with somatoform pain disorder typically has difficulty controlling anxiety. Relaxation techniques can help alleviate anxiety, thereby enabling the client to regain control.*

Evaluation

- Mr. Cruz maintains his weight and reports being able to sleep through the night.
- Although Mr. Cruz still lacks insight into the specific cause of his illness, he engages in ongoing psychotherapy with a clinical nurse specialist.
- Mr. Cruz attends physical therapy once a week.
- Mrs. Cruz sees a clinical nurse specialist to help her cope effectively with her husband's condition.

18 Psychiatric therapies

I. Overview

    A. Health care professionals use various therapies to treat psychiatric disorders

    B. The client may be involved in a single therapeutic modality or a combination of treatment approaches, such as individual, group, family, milieu, and electroconvulsive therapy

    C. Psychiatric theoretical models discussed earlier in this book are utilized in each therapeutic approach; for example, individual psychotherapy can utilize crisis intervention theory, Peplau's concepts of anxiety, and behavioral theory; and group and family therapy can integrate the psychoanalytic model and communication theory

    D. The client's needs and the therapist's skills determine the treatment modality used

II. Individual therapies

    A. Gestalt therapy

        1. First developed in the 1940s, Gestalt therapy has personal self-growth as its primary goal

        2. Focusing on self-awareness, the therapist facilitates the client's ability to engage in self-discovery

        3. The therapist points out discrepancies in the client's behavior and thoughts, without interpreting the behavior or thoughts

        4. The client is encouraged to set personal goals in life and to make independent choices

        5. Gestalt therapy is based on several assumptions

            a. Humans naturally strive to grow and satisfy basic needs

            b. Self-awareness is central to meeting those needs

            c. Reality is whatever is happening now

            d. Focusing on the past or looking to the future prevents one from being totally in the present

            e. To be fully empowered, a person must take total responsibility for making choices in life

        6. Gestalt therapy relies on two therapeutic techniques

            a. Empty chair dialogue: using an empty chair, the client is asked to imagine that a significant other or a past experience is in the chair; the client then engages in a "dialogue" with the chair, with the therapist listening, observing, and calling attention to the client's nonverbal communications

  b. Dream discussion: the client recalls a dream and then acts out every character and event in the dream; dreams are considered a spontaneous psychic production containing an existential message

B. Psychoanalysis

  1. Psychoanalysis is a daily process of examining the working of the mind, using free association and dream analysis

  2. The client is instructed to refrain from all activity during the 50-minute session so that all energy is focused on discovering mental content through verbalization

  3. The analyst seeks verbal patterns that provide insight into the client's intrapsychic conflicts

  4. Dreams, fantasies, wishes, fears, and feelings are discussed during the analysis

  5. The analyst interprets the meaning of the dreams, fantasies, wishes, fears, and feelings, both conscious and unconscious, to help the client see the connection between unconscious wishes and conscious behavior

  6. The analyst-client interaction produces *transference* (the strong emotional response that the client develops toward the therapist) and *countertransference* (the analyst's emotional response to the client)

  7. Success of the analysis depends on successful interpretation of the client's mental content

  8. The client gains insight on how to rework unresolved problems and adopt more adaptive solutions

  9. Psychoanalysis is a long-term therapy that requires a major time and financial commitment from the client

C. Transactional analysis

  1. A theoretical communications model as well as a therapy, transactional analysis examines the communications (transactions) occurring between people, attempting to discover how people relate to one another

  2. It is based on several assumptions

  a. People make current life decisions based on past assumptions that are invalid

  b. Present-day life is restricted because of earlier invalid decisions

  c. Developing an awareness of how present-day life has been influenced by past assumptions enables the client to change behavior

  3. The therapist works with the client to analyze the three levels of ego communication

  a. *Complementary transaction level:* a healthy form of communication occurring between the ego states of adult to adult or child to child

      b. *Crossed transaction level:* a nonproductive form of communication between the ego states of adult to child or child to adult

      c. *Ulterior transaction level:* a destructive form of communication during which one person attempts to feel superior to another

    4. During transactional analysis, the client is taught how to identify the ego state from which he or she operates and how to interrupt an automatic tendency to engage in nonproductive or destructive transactions

    5. The goal of therapy is to promote the use of the complementary transaction level to build maximum client growth

D. Rational emotive therapy

    1. This type of therapy attempts to correct maladaptive behavior by changing established patterns of thinking that arise from underlying irrational thoughts, such as "I must be loved by everyone," "A woman without a man is nothing," or "If things go wrong, it's a catastrophe"

    2. Irrational learned responses are culture specific

    3. The therapist's role is to help the client gain three insights

      a. Irrational beliefs cause current misery; people disturb themselves

      b. An irrational belief is reinforced each time it is used

      c. The best way to change an irrational belief is to do something different; talking about it is ineffective

    4. During the sessions, the therapist aggressively points out and challenges the client's irrational thoughts

    5. The goal of rational emotive therapy is to achieve happiness in life by thinking rationally and by accepting one's strengths and weaknesses

E. Reality therapy

    1. Reality therapy focuses on helping the client meet needs by taking effective control over choices in life

    2. It assumes that human behavior is driven by needs; consequently, when one's needs are not satisfied, one experiences pain

    3. People who meet their needs are successful and happy most of the time; those who do not meet their needs experience failure and pain

    4. The client is constantly confronted during therapy with questions that reinforce self-responsibility, such as "What do you want?" or "What do you think is best?"

    5. The therapist refrains from giving advice

F. Individual psychotherapy

    1. This type of therapy establishes a relationship between the therapist and the client in an attempt to understand the client's intrapsychic conflicts

2. Treatment is aimed at maintaining or modifying adaptive patterns and changing parts of the personality structure to build more effective adaptive behaviors

3. Individual psychotherapy uses two major techniques

    a. *Supportive psychotherapy* strengthens the client's inner defenses to help reduce anxiety; especially effective with clients who have a weak ego structure

    b. *Analytic psychotherapy* uses the interpretation of dreams, free association, and transference distortions to uncover intrapsychic conflicts

4. Psychotherapy is most effective when the client's problem is stress related and the client has the capacity to engage, work through, and disengage the treatment process

G. Behavior modification

    1. The therapist uses a five-step approach to change the client's maladaptive behaviors

        a. Using direct observation, the therapist assesses the client for symptoms of behavioral dysfunction (for instance, stuttering, crying, or inappropriate verbalizations, such as expressions of suicide ideation)

        b. The therapist then discusses treatment goals with the client, focusing on specific behaviors that need changing

        c. Next, the therapist assesses the conditions that either promote or minimize these behaviors (behavioral analysis)

        d. The therapist then alters the client's environment to effect changes in the client's behavior

        e. Finally, the therapist observes, documents, and analyzes any behavioral changes that occur, and either continues the treatment as planned or develops alternative treatments

    2. Behavior modification is based on testing one hypothesis, which may lead to another, which also must be tested

    3. Therapists can use several techniques to modify behavior

        a. Systematic desensitization

            (1) The client learns relaxation techniques and new behaviors that can assist in reducing anxiety

            (2) The client learns to tolerate increasing amounts of anxiety

        b. Graded exposure

            (1) The client gradually makes contact with the source of the anxiety

            (2) The client learns that the anxiety-producing object is really harmless

            (3) Eventually, the object no longer arouses intolerable amounts of anxiety

    c. Social skills training

       (1) The therapist rewards the client only for desirable social behaviors

       (2) The therapist uses group role-playing and modeling to teach social skills

       (3) Between sessions, the client must complete homework assignments to practice and reinforce desirable behaviors

    d. Response prevention

       (1) The therapist asks the client to hesitate briefly before responding, in a characteristic way, to a noxious stimulus

       (2) The therapist then models alternative responses to the stimulus

       (3) The client is rewarded for delaying the characteristic response

       (4) Over time, the client learns to tolerate noxious stimuli without immediately resorting to characteristic maladaptive responses

    e. Token economy

       (1) The therapist provides the client with a list of acceptable behaviors to a stimulus, along with the consequences of exhibiting undesirable behaviors

       (2) For each acceptable behavior exhibited, the therapist awards the client a token, which the client can exchange for desired goods

       (3) Over time, the client learns acceptable behaviors

III. Group therapies

  A. Group psychotherapy

    1. This type of therapy is based on the premise that group influence is a powerful vehicle for structuring and reinforcing behavior

    2. It can be a treatment for many disorders that involve erroneous thinking or distortions of mental perceptions

    3. Group psychotherapy emphasizes the examination of interpersonal relationships; as in individual therapy, the client's ego strength determines which therapeutic technique — supportive or analytic — is used

    4. Central concepts of group psychotherapy include the following:

      a. *Content* refers to what is said in the group

      b. *Process* refers to what is done in the group

      c. *Cohesiveness* refers to the sense of belonging that keeps all members in the group

      d. Other important concepts include *transference* and *countertransference* (see II.B.6.) and *resistance* (forestalling the therapeutic process)

5. Dynamics of a group include the following:
   a. *Rank* refers to the position of a member in the group
   b. *Status* refers to the prestige of a member in the group
   c. *Norms* are the group's rules of conduct or standards for appropriate behavior
   d. *Role* refers to the function or part that a member assumes within the group
6. Every group should serve some therapeutic purpose; common purposes among groups in psychotherapy include the following:
   a. Personality reconstruction
   b. Remotivation and reeducation
   c. Support
   d. Problem solving
7. Specialty groups are those consisting of clients with a commonality, such as age, gender, or educational background
8. All groups must be led by a therapist knowledgeable about group dynamics and process

B. Family therapy
   1. Family therapy is directed toward liberating the client from living in an environment in which there is acting out of family anxieties and conflicts
   2. A therapist meets with the family and attempts to focus on the patterns of family interaction, to reveal family secrets and myths, and to examine and make explicit their nonverbal communications
   3. Goals of family therapy are to minimize conflict, to build awareness of others among the members, and to help individual members deal with internal and external destructive processes
   4. Central concepts of family therapy include the following:
      a. *Triangles:* introduction of a third person into an uncomfortable interaction between two family members, to reduce the tension; a triangle can also be formed around an issue, object, or group
      b. *Multi-generational patterns:* process through which behavioral patterns are transmitted from one generation to another; a genogram is used to map out these patterns of interaction and behavior
      c. *Communication:* family interaction is considered in relation to how family members send, receive, and respond to verbal and nonverbal messages
      d. *Family system:* the whole is more than the sum of its parts; the system can be either functional or dysfunctional, based on its level of differentiation
      e. *Differentiation:* measurement of human functioning on a continuum, from a lower level of strong intensity of emotional fusion to an upper level of complete differentiation and emotional autonomy

(1) A person at the lower level has emotions so fused with those of other family members that the person exhibits little emotional autonomy

(2) A person at the upper level is emotionally and intellectually separated from other family members and is more adaptable to and independent of the emotions that surround the family

 f. *Family projection process:* projection of a family problem onto one or more children in the family (a process used by spouses to avoid marital confrontations)

 g. *Sibling position:* the place and role within the family that a child learns and assumes

C. Psychodrama

 1. This type of therapy uses structured and controlled dramatization of a client's problems

 2. The goal is to dramatize emotional problems so they can be reexperienced and examined in a new way

 3. The therapy group provides immediate feedback to the actor (client) so that new learning can occur

 4. Psychodrama can be cathartic in that the client, after reliving past experiences and the emotions they generated, can rework the emotions in the present time to produce a more acceptable response

 5. Psychodrama comprises three phases

  a. Warm-up

   (1) The group decides which issue to explore

   (2) A protagonist (principal actor) is urged to come forward

  b. Action

   (1) The actors discuss the play to be enacted

   (2) The play begins

   (3) The actors spontaneously portray the roles assigned to them

  c. Post-action group sharing

   (1) The group members (actors) discuss personal experiences that the drama has reactivated

   (2) The members integrate their current feelings with those they once had toward the experiences

   (3) They search for new meaning in the awareness they have developed

 6. The techniques used in psychodrama are designed to enhance self-exploration and understanding

 7. Psychodrama can be effective in dealing with interpersonal conflicts, such as marital discord

IV. Rehabilitation therapies

A. Occupational therapy

1. Occupational therapy is the art and science of guiding a client's participation in crafts and related activities to promote recovery from illness and maintain good health

2. Such programs may involve an individual or a group and may be simple or complex; an occupational activities assessment determines the activity level selected for the client

3. Traditional occupational therapy activities include sewing, weaving, clay sculpturing, and the making of wood and leather artifacts; occupational therapists also participate in teaching daily living skills and other rehabilitation therapies, such as pet therapy and plant therapy

B. Art therapy

1. Art therapy is the use of art to help a client express feelings and inner conflicts

2. Besides being a form of treatment, it also can be a diagnostic tool (for instance, the therapist may interpret the symbolism in a client's drawings)

3. Encouraging a client to draw relieves anxiety and aggression in a socially acceptable way

C. Recreational therapy

1. Recreational therapy is the use of controlled and planned physical activity to promote a client's well-being and comfort

2. It is based on the theory that a positive relationship between one's self and the environment contributes to good health

3. The goals are to provide an outlet for energy release, to teach the client how to play, to teach cooperation with others, and to help the client develop leisure-time pursuits

4. Recreational activities may be vigorous (such as dance, basketball, or tennis) or less strenuous (such as checkers or chess)

5. The recreational therapist also identifies community resources that help integrate a discharged client back into society

D. Play therapy

1. Play therapy is the use of play as a means of communicating with mentally disturbed children

2. It assumes that children younger than age 12 can express themselves better through the manipulation of objects (toys) than through words

3. Observing a child at play provides clues about the child's developmental level, style of interaction, and areas of potential psychic conflict

4. Children engage in five types of play

   a. *Exploratory:* the child experiments with different play techniques

   b. *Creative:* the child uses objects creatively

       c. *Diversional:* the child's activities have no purpose, indicating boredom

       d. *Mimetic:* the child attempts to master a skill by observing repetitive activity

       e. *Cathartic:* the play is hard, intense, and without pleasure; activities symbolize underlying stress

5. Play development has three stages

       a. *Solitary (infant to toddler):* the child plays alone, unaware of others in the immediate environment

       b. *Parallel (toddler to school-age child):* the child plays in close proximity to others but not with them

       c. *Cooperative (school-age child and older):* the child participates in organized play with others

6. Play therapy has several benefits

       a. Promotes self-expression and creativity

       b. Discharges tension and aggression

       c. Enables the child to learn techniques for self-pleasure

       d. Fosters trust among those at play

       e. Permits expression of emotionally charged feelings

V. Other psychiatric therapies

    A. Electroconvulsive therapy (ECT)

      1. An electric current passes through electrodes applied to the client's temples to induce a generalized tonic-clonic seizure and unconsciousness

      2. ECT is based on the observation that epileptics are rarely schizophrenic

      3. It is used to treat clients with involutional depression; bipolar disorder, manic phase; and psychotic symptoms when drugs are contraindicated

      4. Nursing interventions for clients undergoing ECT include the following:

       a. Provide nothing by mouth after midnight to prevent vomiting during treatment

       b. Remove all prostheses, including dentures

       c. Dress the client in loose-fitting clothing

       d. Teach the client and family about the treatment and what to expect

       e. Obtain a signed informed consent

       f. Provide close observation immediately after the treatment

       g. Use the same nursing care procedures as for an unconscious client

    B. Psychoeducation

      1. Psychoeducation is the use of educational principles and techniques to rehabilitate and treat psychiatric clients

    2. It is used to teach clients and their families about the client's illness

    3. It fosters collaboration and active participation in the treatment program

    4. Clients who are exposed to psychoeducation learn information that helps them improve the quality of their lives; families learn how to accept and cope with a client's illness, minimizing stress for all concerned

C. Milieu therapy

    1. Milieu therapy aims to treat a mental disorder by manipulating the client's environment and focusing on the atmosphere of treatment

    2. Its effectiveness depends on the attitudes of the health care team and their interaction with the client

    3. Through self-government, the client assumes some responsibility for the management of the unit on which he or she lives

    4. The unit is structured to provide human relationships that satisfy emotional needs, reduce psychological conflicts and deprivation, and strengthen impaired ego functions

    5. Characteristics of a therapeutic milieu include the following:

        a. The client and staff share responsibility for care, including such issues as passes, discharges, and status changes

        b. Role relationships are examined to determine which behaviors are appropriate

        c. Staff members have ultimate authority for making decisions and establishing policies

        d. Socialization and group interaction are emphasized in order to provide the best opportunity for living and learning

    6. The primary goal of milieu therapy is to provide an atmosphere in which the client can learn to live a productive and successful life in society

    7. The nurse's role is a central component of milieu therapy because nurses are present on the unit 24 hours a day

19

Psychopharmacology

I. Overview

    A. Before the early 1950s, the care of mentally ill persons consisted primarily of removing them from families and loved ones and placing them indefinitely in extremely crowded institutions, where treatment may or may not have been provided

        1. Crude treatment modalities — such as insulin shock therapy; electroconvulsive therapy; frontal lobe lobotomy; and the use of "cold packs," straight jackets, and padded cells — were the only "therapeutic interventions" available to treat symptoms of psychosis and depression

        2. The history of how these interventions were administered on such a vulnerable population contains documented evidence of inhumane attitudes and physical abuse, a legacy that today haunts not only the field of psychiatry and its practitioners but also those seeking treatment for mental distress

    B. A milestone in the treatment of mental disorders occurred with the introduction of chlorpromazine (Thorazine) to therapeutic regimens

        1. The drug, discovered in France in the early 1950s, was initially used in the treatment of manic disorders

        2. Clinicians noted calmness, marked indifference to surroundings, and lowered body temperature in clients who received it

        3. In 1955, clinicians in the United States began administering the drug to clients with psychotic and schizophrenic symptoms, particularly to those who exhibited violent behavior

        4. Clinicians observed significant improvement among such clients, as evidenced by a notable decline in violent and unruly behavior

    C. Such behavioral improvements heightened the concerns of families and, eventually, politicians, that institutionalization was preventing many humans from living to their fullest potential

    D. The Joint Commission on Mental Health and Mental Illness prompted the establishment of the federal Community Mental Health Centers Act, which was passed in 1963

        1. Under that law, President Kennedy proposed a "bold new approach" to the treatment of mental disorders, one that emphasized returning hospitalized clients to active rehabilitation services in the community

Managing the adverse effects of psychotropic agents

Although psychotropic agents can dramatically improve the health status of a client with a psychiatric problem, their adverse effects can produce problems for the client. These may range from minor discomforts, such as dry mouth, to more serious conditions, such as tardive dyskinesia and neuroleptic malignant syndrome. The following chart presents common adverse effects of psychotropic agents, along with appropriate nursing interventions.

ADVERSE EFFECTS	NURSING INTERVENTIONS
Drowsiness, dizziness, hypotension, blurred vision, faulty reflexes and perceptions	• Advise the client to rise slowly, hold on to furniture, and avoid slippery or cluttered floors. • Warn the client that the drug may interfere with driving ability, especially at the beginning of therapy. • Check the client's blood pressure in prone and standing positions.
Dry mouth	• Offer the client mints, ice chips, or chewing gum. • Advise the client to hold fluids in the mouth momentarily before swallowing. • Apply petrolatum to the client's lips.
Nasal stuffiness	• Add humidity to the room by using a steam vaporizer.
Weight gain	• Encourage the client to follow a low-calorie diet and to exercise within limits.
Constipation	• Ensure an adequate amount of bulk and fluids in the client's diet. • Promote regular exercise. • Establish regular times for elimination; use a mild laxative, if needed.
Libido changes	• Explain that psychotropic agents sometimes produce temporary changes in libido. • Reassure the client that sexual drive will eventually return to normal.
Photosensitivity, pruritus, grayish-purple skin discoloration	• Caution the client to apply sunscreen and to wear sunglasses and protective clothing when outdoors; direct sunlight intensifies skin rash and discoloration. • Suggest that the client use lotion to relieve itching.
Blood dyscrasia (agranulocytosis)	• Teach the client to report fever, sore throat, unusual malaise, or infection (such as vaginitis, dermatitis, or gastritis). • Have complete blood count (CBC) and differential studies performed to establish baseline data; then have the studies performed periodically. (If the client is taking clozapine, weekly CBCs are necessary.) • Consult the physician about decreasing the dosage.
Jaundice or liver damage	• Inform the client that prolonged treatment or high dosage may decrease liver function. • Teach the family to observe for yellowish sclera or skin. • Have liver function tests performed occasionally.
Extrapyramidal reactions (secondary parkinsonism); akathisia; rigid limbs and drooling; tremors of hands and limbs; taut skin, unsteady gait, and posture changes; akinesia, weakness, fatigue, painful limbs (occurs most commonly in people between ages 15 and 18, in elderly persons, and in women)	• Reduce the dosage, as prescribed (antiparkinsonian drugs are usually ordered). • Promote safety measures. • Modify care and activities so the client can maintain self-esteem. • Assist the client, as needed, with eating, hygiene, grooming, and mobility.

(continued)

Managing the adverse effects of psychotropic agents *(continued)*

ADVERSE EFFECTS	NURSING INTERVENTIONS
Tardive dyskinesia (with chronic use of antipsychotics)	• Assess the client frequently by using the Abnormal Involuntary Movement Scale (AIMS examination). • Report abnormalities to the prescribing physician or nurse practitioner.
Neuroleptic malignant syndrome	• Monitor the client regularly for temperature elevation. • Assess the client's mental status if the temperature rises quickly. • If the client demonstrates changes in mental status, such as delirium or confusion, notify the prescribing physician immediately, discontinue the drug, and seek emergency medical treatment.

    2. This proposal, which sparked what became known as the "Deinstitutionalization Movement," was made possible by the advent of medications for the treatment of mental disorders

  E. Other advancements in science and technology have paved the way for continued improvements in treatment

    1. Greater understanding of the complexities of brain functioning and its relationship to psychiatric illness and modern therapy led scientists to recognize the significance of dopamine receptors and their effects on psychosis; this discovery challenged the traditional psychodynamic view of "poor nurturing" as being the sole cause of mental illness

    2. Sophisticated technology, such as positron emission tomography (PET), has allowed scientists to examine brain physiology and neurochemical actions in human beings

      a. Increased density of dopamine receptors in nontreated schizophrenics has been observed through the use of the PET scan

      b. These findings show a direct correlation between neurochemical actions in the brain and the role they play in psychiatric illness

  F. Although they can provide symptom relief, psychotropic medications are not a cure for mental illness; they should always be used as an adjunct to other psychotherapeutic interventions

II. Antipsychotic agents

  A. Indications

    1. Acute and chronic psychosis associated with depression or schizophrenia

    2. Bipolar disorder, manic phase

    3. Paranoia

    4. Severe nausea and vomiting (antiemetic)

    5. Control of tics associated with Tourette's syndrome

B. Mechanism of action
   1. Block dopamine receptors in the central nervous system (basal gan-glia, limbic system, hypothalamus, brain stem, and medulla), thereby reducing psychotic symptoms
   2. Block adrenergic and muscarinic receptors and exert an effect on other transmitters, such as gamma-aminobutyric acid (GABA), and peptides

C. Absorption, distribution, and elimination
   1. Most antipsychotic medications are available in tablet, syrup, and in-jectable forms
      a. Liquid preparations are absorbed more rapidly than tablets
      b. Parenteral administration is absorbed rapidly, with the initial drug effect occurring within 15 minutes; peak plasma level oc-curs within 60 minutes
      c. Depot preparations are long-acting antipsychotic medications given intramuscularly in an oily preparation that slows the ab-sorption rate; three preparations are available: fluphenazine decanoate, fluphenazine enanthate, and haloperidol
   2. Oral drugs usually are distributed adequately, although food or antac-ids may decrease their absorption
   3. Drugs are metabolized in the liver and kidneys and excreted through the kidneys, enterohepatic circulation, and feces
   4. Excretion is slow; metabolites may be found in urine up to 6 months after drug discontinuation

D. Adverse effects
   1. Acute dystonic reactions
      a. Muscle spasms of the tongue, face, neck, or back
      b. Possible oculogyric crisis, usually within the first 5 days of treat-ment
      c. Treatment: antihistamines or anticholinergic drugs
   2. Akathisia
      a. Motor restlessness that is commonly mistaken for psychotic rest-lessness or agitation
      b. May appear after the first few days of treatment
      c. Symptoms: difficulty in sitting; pacing, fidgeting, constant move-ment of extremities
      d. Treatment: dosage reduction or different medication; muscle re-laxants sometimes helpful
   3. Secondary parkinsonism
      a. Motor retardation and rigidity
      b. Difficulty in initiating or carrying out motor activity
      c. Shuffling gait
      d. Hypersalivation
      e. Tremors in the hands and legs

Profile of antipsychotic agents

Antipsychotic agents comprise six chemical classes that produce adverse effects of varying intensity. Low-potency agents tend to exert greater sedative and anticholinergic effects and to cause more postural hypotension. High-potency agents tend to produce more extrapyramidal adverse effects.

The following chart lists generic and trade names, daily dosages, and major effects of representative drugs from each chemical class. (Classes appear in boldface type; subclasses appear in italic type.)

DRUG	DAILY DOSAGE	ADVERSE EFFECTS
Phenothiazines		
Aliphatics chlorpromazine (Thorazine)	30 to 800 mg	• High sedative and hypotensive effects • Medium anticholinergic effect • Low extrapyramidal effects
triflupromazine (Vesprin)	60 to 150 mg	• High sedative and hypotensive effects • Medium anticholinergic and extrapyramidal effects
Piperidines mesoridazine (Serentil)	100 to 400 mg	• Medium sedative, hypotensive, anticholinergic, and extrapyramidal effects
thioridazine (Mellaril)	30 to 800 mg	• High sedative, hypotensive, and anticholinergic effects • Low extrapyramidal effects
Piperazines acetophenazine (Tindal)	40 to 80 mg	• Low sedative, hypotensive, and anticholinergic effects • Medium extrapyramidal effects
fluphenazine (Prolixin)	1 to 20 mg	• Medium sedative effects • Low hypotensive and anticholinergic effects • High extrapyramidal effects
perphenazine (Trilafon)	6 to 64 mg	• Low sedative, hypotensive, and anticholinergic effects • High extrapyramidal effects
trifluoperazine (Stelazine)	2 to 20 mg	• Medium sedative effects • Low hypotensive and anticholinergic effects • High extrapyramidal effects
Thioxanthenes		
Aliphatic chlorprothixene (Taractan)	25 to 600 mg	• High sedative, hypotensive, and anticholinergic effects • Low extrapyramidal effects

Profile of antipsychotic agents *(continued)*

DRUG	DAILY DOSAGE	ADVERSE EFFECTS
Piperazine thiothixene (Navane)	6 to 60 mg	• Low sedative, hypotensive, and anticholinergic effects • High extrapyramidal effects
Dibenzoxazepine		
loxapine (Loxitane)	20 to 250 mg	• Medium sedative, hypotensive, and anticholinergic effects • High extrapyramidal effects
Butyrophenone		
haloperidol (Haldol)	4 to 60 mg	• Low sedative, hypotensive, and anticholinergic effects • High extrapyramidal effects
Dihydroindolone		
molindone (Moban)	5 to 150 mg	• Medium sedative and anticholinergic effects • Low hypotensive effects • High extrapyramidal effects
Dibenzodiazepine		
clozapine (Clozaril)	300 to 450 mg	• Low sedative, hypotensive, anticholinergic, and extrapyramidal effects

    f. Treatment: anticholinergic medication and dosage reduction

  4. Tardive dyskinesia

    a. Potential permanent complication of long-term neuroleptic drug therapy, believed to result from the development of receptors that are supersensitive to dopamine after prolonged blockade

    b. Common symptoms

      (1) Excessive facial movements (including grimacing, blinking, and ticlike movements, particularly around the mouth)

      (2) Protrusion of the tongue (sometimes called "fly catcher" tongue), puffing of the cheeks or the tongue in the cheek

      (3) Thrusting of extremities and neck

      (4) Involuntary, usually choreoathetoid movements

    c. Treatment: dosage reduction or medication discontinuation

  5. Neuroleptic malignant syndrome

    a. Rare, life-threatening reaction to neuroleptic drugs, especially high-potency drugs

    b. Causes hyperthermia, rigidity, impaired consciousness, unstable automatic functions, hypertension, hypotension, elevated white blood cell count and creatinine phosphokinase (CPK) level, and cardiac arrhythmias

      c. Treatment: immediate discontinuation of the drug, cooling blankets, restoration of hydration and fluid and electrolyte balances, administration of dantrolene sodium and bromocriptine mesylate

  6. Other possible effects

    a. Breathing difficulty

    b. Uncontrollable hypersalivation

    c. Grunting

    d. Sedation

    e. Hypotension

    f. Changes in ECG T waves

    g. Lowered seizure threshold

    h. Endocrine disturbances

      (1) Increased prolactin levels from dopamine blockade

      (2) Amenorrhea

    i. Weight gain

    j. Changes in libido

    k. Photosensitivity

    l. Cholestatic hepatitis

    m. Blood dyscrasias, including aplastic anemia

    n. Anticholinergic effects

      (1) Dry mouth

      (2) Blurred vision

      (3) Constipation

      (4) Urine retention

    o. Treatment: dosage reduction or medication discontinuation

E. Contraindications

  1. Known hypersensitivity

  2. Comatose states

  3. Use in combination with known central nervous system (CNS) depressants, such as alcohol, narcotics, and barbiturates

  4. Blood dyscrasias

  5. Liver, renal, or cardiac dysfunctions

F. Nursing considerations

  1. Ensure that the client undergoes a thorough physiologic and psychological assessment before taking an antipsychotic medication; include family members or significant others in the assessment so they can be informed of drug interactions and potential adverse effects

  2. Document all client and family teaching

  3. Encourage the client to practice sound health habits and to undergo a yearly physical examination

4. Tell the client to report adverse reactions or discomfort from the medication

5. Be aware that safety for use in pregnancy has not been established; precautions should be taken, particularly during the first trimester

6. Know that antipsychotic drugs are excreted in breast milk

III. Antiparkinsonian agents

A. Indication: to relieve the neurologic adverse effects of antipsychotic drugs

B. Mechanism of action: block central cholinergic receptors

C. Absorption, distribution, and elimination
  1. Variable absorption in the GI tract
  2. Cross the blood-brain barrier
  3. Eliminated in urine and feces

D. Adverse effects
  1. Anticholinergic
    a. Dry mouth
    b. Constipation
    c. Blurred vision
    d. Urine retention
    e. Flushed skin
  2. Gastrointestinal
    a. Nausea
    b. Vomiting
  3. Central nervous system
    a. Impaired cognitive functioning
    b. Disorientation
    c. Confusion
    d. Hallucinations
    e. Restlessness
    f. Weakness
  4. Other
    a. Suppression of sweating, causing hyperthermia
    b. Toxic psychosis, with symptoms of euphoria, confusion, and disorientation

E. Contraindications
  1. Prostatic hypertrophy
  2. Anuria
  3. Acute angle-closure glaucoma

Common antiparkinsonian agents

The chart below lists the usual daily adult dosages for and primary effects of the most commonly administered antiparkinsonian agents.

DRUG	DAILY DOSAGE	EFFECTS
benztropine (Cogentin)	Initial dose: 1 to 2 mg I.M. or I.V.; may repeat in 30 minutes. Maintenance dose: 1 to 6 mg	Acts as muscle relaxant, reduces rigidity and drooling, relieves dystonic reactions, exerts sedative actions.
trihexyphenidyl (Artane)	4 to 15 mg	Exerts mild effect on rigidity and spasms, alleviates tremors; administered during the day for lethargic and akinetic clients.
biperiden (Akineton)	2 to 8 mg	Reduces rigidity and akinesia.
amantadine (Symmetrel)	100 to 400 mg	Improves akathisia, akinesia, dystonias, secondary parkinsonism, and rigidity; however, tolerance to dosage may develop after 2 to 3 weeks.

F. Nursing considerations

1. Teach the client the proper use of antiparkinsonian agents; instruct the client not to increase the dosage without consulting the physician

2. Monitor the client's intake and output to assess for urine retention (especially in an elderly client)

3. Observe the client for signs of toxicity

4. Administer medications after meals to avoid gastric irritation

5. Instruct the client to relieve dry mouth with sugarless gum or candy

6. Teach the client to prevent weight gain by avoiding high-calorie drinks and sweets

7. Be aware of the possible association between use of anticholinergic agents and minor fetal malformations; if possible, the client should avoid taking the drug during the first trimester of pregnancy

8. Caution the client about breast-feeding while taking these drugs (no supportive data available)

IV. Tricyclic antidepressants

A. Indications

1. Depressive disorders

2. Psychotic depression

3. Attention deficit disorder

    4. Obsessive-compulsive disorder

    5. Organic affective disorder

    6. Bulimia

    7. Post-traumatic stress disorder

    8. Neurogenic pain syndromes

    9. Migraine headaches

    10. Enuresis in children and adolescents

B. Mechanism of action: unknown (drugs may block the reuptake of norepinephrine and serotonin to their presynaptic state, increasing the concentration of these neurotransmitters)

C. Absorption, distribution, and elimination

    1. Absorbed in the GI tract

    2. Binds to plasma and tissue protein

    3. Highly lipophilic, metabolized in the liver, with nonlipophilic metabolites being excreted in feces and urine

D. Adverse effects

    1. Allergic: rash

    2. Anticholinergic

        a. Blurred vision

        b. Dry mouth

        c. Constipation

        d. Urine retention

        e. Increased perspiration

        f. Speech difficulty

        g. Mental clouding, confusion, and delirium

    3. Cardiovascular

        a. Postural hypotension

        b. Dizziness

        c. Hypertension

        d. Sinus tachycardia

        e. Premature atrial or ventricular beats

        f. Myocardial depression

        g. Pedal edema

        h. Worsening of congestive heart failure

        i. ECG changes

            (1) Depressed ST segment

            (2) Flat or inverted T wave

            (3) Prolonged QRS complex

    4. Gastrointestinal

        a. Nausea

        b. Vomiting

        c. Heartburn

5. Neurologic
   a. Drowsiness
   b. Muscle tremors, twitches
   c. Nervousness
   d. Paresthesia
   e. Fatigue, weakness
   f. Ataxia
   g. Seizures (with overdose or in a client with a known seizure disorder, hallucinations, delusions, or activation of schizophrenic or manic psychoses)
6. Overdose and toxicity
   a. Average lethal dose: adults, 30 mg/kg of body weight; children, 20 mg/kg of body weight
   b. Initial symptoms: fever, irritability, confusion, hallucinations, delirium, hypertension, and choreiform movements
   c. Late symptoms: cardiac abnormalities, drowsiness, respiratory depression, cyanosis, congestive heart failure, and shock
   d. Treatment of overdose: hospitalization, with close monitoring of cardiovascular and respiratory systems; removal of drug from the stomach by lavage and administration of activated charcoal

E. Contraindications
   1. Excessive use of alcohol and sedatives
   2. History of seizures or suicide attempts
   3. Urine retention
   4. Acute angle-closure glaucoma
   5. Hypersensitivity to the drug
   6. Acute recovery phase of myocardial infarction
   7. Concomitant use of MAO inhibitors (usually)

F. Nursing considerations
   1. Teach the client the proper use of medications, and explain adverse effects
      a. Instruct the client to take medications at night to prevent daytime drowsiness and dizziness
      b. Reassure the client that these symptoms will decrease in 2 to 3 weeks
   2. Monitor the client's behavior for early adverse effects of the medications
   3. Observe for increased psychomotor activity
   4. Assess the client's suicide potential
   5. Instruct the client to report urine retention
   6. Teach the client the importance of following a proper diet, with emphasis on increasing roughage and bulk to prevent constipation
   7. Take measures to prevent or minimize dry mouth

Common antidepressant agents

In treating a client with depression, the physician may prescribe a tricyclic or atypical antidepressant or a monoamine oxidase (MAO) inhibitor. The following chart presents the usual adult daily dosage of commonly administered antidepressant agents, along with the intensity of their sedative and anticholinergic effects. Drugs for elderly clients usually should be administered in divided doses, with the maximum dosage being half the recommended adult dosage, unless stated otherwise.

DRUG	DAILY DOSAGE	SEDATIVE EFFECTS	ANTICHOLINERGIC EFFECTS
Tricyclic antidepressants			
amitriptyline (Elavil, Endep)	10 to 50 mg (elderly clients) 150 to 300 mg (adult clients)	High	High
desipramine (Norpramin, Pertofrane)	25 to 100 mg (elderly clients)	Low	Low
doxepin (Adapin, Sinequan)	25 to 50 mg (elderly clients) 150 to 300 mg (adult clients)	High	High
imipramine (Tofranil, Janimine)	150 to 300 mg	Low	High
trimipramine (Surmontil)	75 mg (elderly clients) 150 to 300 mg (adult clients)	High	Moderate
nortriptyline (Aventyl, Pamelor)	75 to 150 mg	Low	Moderate
protriptyline (Vivactil)	15 mg (elderly clients) 10 to 60 mg (adult clients)	Low	Moderate
amoxapine (Asendin)	100 to 400 mg	Low	Low
maprotiline (Ludiomil)	150 to 300 mg	High	Low
Atypical antidepressants			
trazodone (Desyrel)	100 to 600 mg	High	Low
fluoxetine (Prozac)	40 to 80 mg	Low	Low
sertraline (Zoloft)	50 to 200 mg	Low	Low
bupropion (Wellbutrin)	225 to 450 mg	Low	Low
MAO inhibitors			
isocarboxazid (Marplan)	30 to 50 mg	Low	Low
phenelzine (Nardil)	45 to 90 mg	Low	Low
tranylcypromine (Parnate)	20 to 60 mg	Low	Low

      a. Offer sugarless candy and gum

      b. Encourage the client to increase fluid intake; offer sugarless drinks to prevent weight gain

  8. Know that psychotherapy will be used in conjunction with drug therapy to treat a client with depression

  9. Be aware that tricyclic antidepressants should be avoided in the first trimester of pregnancy and that they are excreted in breast milk (Note: they have not been proven to have teratogenic effects)

V. Monoamine oxidase (MAO) inhibitors

A. Indication: symptomatic treatment of depression, especially atypical depression

B. Mechanism of action: inhibit the action of the enzyme monoamine oxidase, thereby preventing the degradation of norepinephrine and serotonin and increasing their concentration in nerve tissue, liver, and lungs

C. Absorption, distribution, and elimination

  1. Absorbed in the GI tract

  2. Metabolized in the liver and excreted by the kidneys

D. Adverse effects

  1. Anticholinergic (most common)

      a. Blurred vision

      b. Dry mouth

      c. Constipation

      d. Urine retention

      e. Increased perspiration

      f. Speech difficulty

      g. Mental clouding, confusion, and delirium

  2. Insomnia and restlessness

  3. Hypomania in clients with bipolar disorder

  4. Myoclonic jerks during sleep

  5. Hypertensive crisis

      a. May occur after the client ingests food that contains tyramine or takes a drug with sympathomimetic properties (many over-the-counter drugs fit this description)

      b. Can be life threatening if not treated (discontinuation of the drug; I.V. administration of phentolamine 5 mg, an alpha-receptor antagonist that will lower the client's blood pressure)

E. Contraindications

  1. Renal or liver disease

  2. Hypertension

  3. Cardiac arrhythmias

  4. Epilepsy

  5. Parkinsonism

F. Nursing considerations

1. Teach the client the proper use of prescribed medications, and explain their adverse effects

2. Advise the client to take these medications early in the day to avoid insomnia

3. Caution the client to avoid over-the-counter cold remedies, decongestants (including nasal sprays and drops), antihistamines, sleep aids, stimulants, and appetite suppressants

4. Instruct the client to avoid foods that contain high levels of tyramine (aged cheese, meat extracts, pickled herring, sour cream and yogurt, soy sauce, chocolate, dried fruits, sausage, salami, pepperoni, bologna, red wine, beer, sherry, caviar, snails, and fermented foods)

5. Educate the client about possible hypotension; demonstrate how to rise slowly from a chair or bed

6. Urge the client to report unexpected symptoms, such as headaches or increased palpitations

VI. Antimanic agents

A. Indication: treatment of bipolar disorder

B. Mechanism of action: unknown (lithium competes with sodium and other cations, thereby affecting the activity of the nerve cell)

C. Absorption, distribution, and elimination

1. Absorbed in the GI tract

2. Distributed throughout all body tissues, including spinal fluid and breast milk; cross the placental barrier

3. Not metabolized; about 95% excreted in urine

D. Adverse effects

1. Gastrointestinal

   a. Irritation

   b. Nausea

   c. Vomiting

   d. Diarrhea

2. Neurologic

   a. Fine tremor of hand (most common at higher dosages; relieved when medication is discontinued)

   b. Fatigue

   c. Nervousness

3. Renal: polyuria

4. Endocrine: hypothyroidism

5. Toxicity

   a. Mild: can develop gradually over several days

Agents commonly used to treat mania

The following chart presents the half-life, usual daily dosage, and recommended serum level for agents commonly administered in the treatment of mania. Among these agents are the anticonvulsants carbamazepine and valproic acid.

DRUG	DAILY DOSAGE	HALF-LIFE	RECOMMENDED SERUM LEVEL
lithium carbonate (Eskalith, Lithane, Lithizine, Lithonate, Lithotabs)	900 to 2,400 mg (acute) 600 to 1,200 mg (maintenance)	8 to 35 hours	0.8 to 1.2 mEq/liter (acute) 0.6 to 1.1 mEq/liter (maintenance)
carbamazepine (Tegretol)	300 to 1,200 mg	16 to 24 hours	17 to 54 mmol/liter
valproic acid	750 to 3,000 mg	6 to 16 hours	350 to 700 mmol/liter

      (1) Symptoms: ataxia, confusion, diarrhea, drowsiness, and slurred speech

      (2) Treatment: discontinuation of lithium

  b. Severe: can occur when drug levels exceed 1.5 to 2 mEq/liter

      (1) Symptom: coma

      (2) Treatment: restoration of fluid and electrolyte balance; hemodialysis (more effective) or peritoneal dialysis

E. Contraindications

  1. Cardiovascular disease

  2. Renal disease

  3. Liver disease

  4. Organic brain damage

  5. Pregnancy

F. Nursing considerations

  1. Teach the client and family the proper use of prescribed medications, and explain interactions and adverse effects

  2. Carefully monitor serum drug levels when the client begins taking the medication

  3. Observe for signs and symptoms of toxicity

  4. Instruct the client to report adverse effects of medications

  5. Urge the client not to self-medicate, particularly with diuretics

  6. Encourage the client to increase fluid intake (while avoiding drinks with sugar and caffeine)

7. Instruct the client to report dietary changes, particularly those involving low-sodium diets

8. Explain the importance of regular laboratory monitoring (serum drug levels, kidney and thyroid functions, hematology studies)

9. Remember that congenital defects have been reported with use during pregnancy

10. Be aware that the drug is excreted in breast milk and that breast-feeding should be discouraged

VII. Benzodiazepines

A. Indications

1. Anxiety

2. Insomnia

3. Alcohol withdrawal syndrome

4. Bipolar disorder, manic phase (in conjunction with lithium)

5. Seizures

B. Mechanism of action: depress the CNS at the limbic system, the brain reticular system, and the cerebral cortex

C. Absorption, distribution, and elimination

1. Well absorbed in the GI tract (although food can delay the rate of absorption)

2. Distribution and elimination possibly influenced by physical disorders (such as liver disease), smoking, age, and use of other drugs

3. Found throughout all body tissues and breast milk; cross the placental barrier

4. Metabolized by the liver and excreted in urine

D. Adverse effects

1. Central nervous system

   a. Depression

   b. Fatigue

   c. Drowsiness

   d. Nystagmus

   e. Muscle weakness

   f. Dysarthria

   g. Ataxia

2. Anticholinergic

   a. Blurred vision

   b. Confusion

   c. Disorientation (primarily in elderly clients)

3. Other effects

   a. Paradoxical agitation, rage reactions, insomnia, nightmares, and hallucinations in clients with a history of violent or aggressive behavior

Selected benzodiazepines

The chart below lists the usual adult daily dosage, half-life, and primary uses of commonly administered benzodiazepines. Note that dosages for elderly clients should be half the dosages given here.

DRUG	DAILY DOSAGE	HALF-LIFE	PRIMARY USES
Short-acting			
triazolam (Halcion)	0.25 to 2 mg	1.5 to 5.5 hours	Hypnotic
Intermediate			
alprazolam (Xanax)	0.25 to 4 mg	12 to 15 hours	Anxiolytic; sedative; treatment of alcohol withdrawal syndrome, depression with anxiety, and panic attacks
halazepam (Paxipam)	1 to 10 mg	14 hours	Anxiolytic; hypnotic
lorazepam (Ativan)	1 to 10 mg	10 to 20 hours	Anxiolytic; preoperative sedation; treatment of alcohol withdrawal syndrome, catatonia, and akathisia
oxazepam (Serax)	30 to 120 mg	5 to 20 hours	Anxiolytic; sedative; treatment of alcohol withdrawal syndrome; reduction of aggression in hostile clients
temazepam (Restoril)	30 mg	10 to 17 hours	Sedative; hypnotic
Long-acting			
chlordiazepoxide (Librium)	25 mg	5 to 30 hours	Anxiolytic; sedative; treatment of alcohol withdrawal syndrome
clonazepam (Klonopin)	0.25 to 2 mg	18 to 50 hours	Anticonvulsant; anxiolytic; treatment of panic attacks and akathisia
clorazepate (Tranxene)	10 to 60 mg	30 to 100 hours	Anxiolytic; treatment of alcohol withdrawal syndrome; adjunct therapy for seizures
diazepam (Valium)	2 to 20 mg	20 to 80 hours	Anxiolytic; anticonvulsant; muscle relaxant; preoperative sedation; treatment of akithisia
flurazepam (Dalmane)	15 to 30 mg	50 to 100 hours	Hypnotic
prazepam (Centrax)	10 mg	30 to 100 hours	Anxiolytic

         b. Respiratory depression from high dosages

         c. Toxicity

            (1) Rarely fatal if taken alone

            (2) Can be fatal in combination with other CNS depressants, such as alcohol and barbiturates

            (3) Symptoms of overdose: depressed respirations, hypertension, and coma

E. Contraindications

    1. Sleep apnea

    2. Liver disease

    3. History of alcohol or drug abuse

F. Nursing considerations

    1. Teach the client the proper use of prescribed medications, and explain their adverse effects

    2. Caution the client not to use the drug in combination with other CNS depressants, such as alcohol and barbiturates

    3. Warn the client not to adjust the dosage without consulting the physician, and explain that tolerance may develop with chronic use

    4. Advise the client to avoid caffeine, which would counteract the effects of the prescribed medication

    5. Caution the client not to drive a car or operate machinery while taking the medication, because mental alertness may be impaired

    6. Continue to assess the client's response to the medication

        a. Determine if target symptoms are being treated

        b. Assess whether oversedation has occurred (particularly with an elderly client)

VIII. Sedative-hypnotics

A. Indications

    1. Anxiety (barbiturates are seldom used as anxiolytics because of their potential for tolerance, dependence, and toxicity; antihistamines are sometimes used as anxiolytics in pediatric and elderly clients)

    2. Insomnia (chloral hydrate derivatives)

    3. Prevention of alcohol withdrawal symptoms (chloral hydrate derivatives)

B. Mechanism of action

    1. Barbiturates: suppress the reticular activating formation of the midbrain, resulting in sedation, sleep, and anesthesia

    2. Antihistamines: compete with histamine for H_1 receptor sites on effector cells

    3. Chloral hydrate derivatives: not fully understood

C. Absorption, distribution, and elimination

1. Barbiturates: absorbed in the GI tract; metabolized in the liver; excreted in urine
2. Antihistamines: absorbed in the GI tract but only 40% to 60% enters the systemic circulation; metabolized in the liver; excreted in urine
3. Chloral hydrate derivatives: absorbed in the GI tract or rectal mucosa; metabolized in the liver; excreted by the kidneys and through bile in feces

D. Adverse effects
1. Barbiturates
   a. Dependence with long-term use
   b. Symptoms of toxicity with long-term use
      (1) Excitement
      (2) Restlessness
      (3) Delirium
      (4) Ataxia
      (5) Nystagmus
      (6) Stupor
      (7) Hypothermia
2. Antihistamines: have few adverse effects
3. Chloral hydrate derivatives
   a. Dependence with use after several weeks
   b. Symptoms of toxicity with long-term use
      (1) Incoordination
      (2) Slurred speech
      (3) Fatigue
      (4) Tremors
      (5) Possible coma, respiratory depression, and cardiac dysfunction

E. Contraindications
1. Previous addiction
2. Liver of kidney impairment
3. Respiratory disease
4. Hypersensitivity

F. Nursing considerations
1. Teach the client the proper use of prescribed medications, and explain their adverse effects
2. Warn the client not to adjust the dosage without consulting the physician
3. Caution the client about the potential for tolerance and dependence with chronic use
4. Inform the client that continued use may worsen sleep patterns

Selected sedative-hypnotics

The chart below lists the usual adult daily dosage, half-life, and primary uses of commonly prescribed sedative-hypnotics.

DRUG	DAILY DOSAGE	HALF-LIFE	PRIMARY USES
Antihistamines			
diphenhydramine (Benadryl)	25 to 50 mg	3 to 4 hours	Hypnotic; anxiolytic
doxylamine (Unisom)	25 mg	10 hours	Hypnotic
hydroxyzine (Atarax)	25 to 100 mg	3 hours	Anxiolytic; hypnotic; sedative
Barbiturates			
amobarbital (Amytal)	65 to 200 mg	20 hours	Hypnotic; also used as a diagnostic aid in hysteria
pentobarbital (Nembutal)	50 to 200 mg	35 to 50 hours	Hypnotic; preoperative sedation
secobarbital (Seconal)	50 to 200 mg	35 to 50 hours	Hypnotic; preoperative sedation
Chloral hydrate derivatives			
chloral hydrate (Noctec)	500 mg to 1 g	8 to 10 hours	Hypnotic

5. Suggest alternative methods of treating insomnia
   a. Avoid caffeine if possible during the day, and particularly after 6 p.m.
   b. Drink herbal teas
6. Encourage the client to refrain from daytime naps and to follow a daily routine that incorporates exercise and relaxation techniques

Post-test

This post-test has been designed to evaluate your readiness to take the certification examination for psychiatric and mental health nursing. Similar in form and content to the actual examination, the post-test consists of 60 questions based on brief clinical situations; the questions will help sharpen your test-taking skills while assessing your knowledge of psychiatric and mental health nursing theory and practice.

You will have 60 minutes to complete the post-test. To improve your chances of performing well, consider these suggestions:

• Read each clinical situation and question attentively; weigh the four options carefully; then select the option that best answers the question. (*Note:* In this post-test, options are lettered A, B, C, and D to aid in later identification of the correct answers and rationales. These letters will not appear in the certification examination.)

• Completely darken the circle in front of the answer that you select, using a #2 pencil (you must use a #2 pencil when taking the certification examination). Do not use check marks, Xs, or lines.

• If you decide to change your answer, erase the old answer completely. (The certification examination is scored electronically; an incomplete erasure may cause both answers to be scored, in which case you will not receive credit for answering the question.)

• If you have difficulty understanding a question or are not sure of the answer, place a small mark next to the question number and, if time permits, come back to it later. If you have no idea of the correct answer, make an educated guess. (Only correct answers are counted in scoring the certification examination, so guessing is preferable to leaving a question unanswered.)

After you have completed the post-test, or the 60-minute time limit expires, check your responses against the correct answers and rationales provided on pages 216 to 229.

Now, select a quiet room where you will be undisturbed, set a timer for 60 minutes, and begin.

1. A nurse enters the dayroom and observes a rather buxom client sitting at a table, playing cards with two male clients. The client is wearing designer boots, a calf-length skirt, and a colorful vest over her otherwise bare chest. What is the nurse's *best* response to this client?

   ○ A. "You need to go to your room and finish dressing."

   ○ B. "It is not proper for you to be wearing only a vest."

   ○ C. "Where are your blouse, slip, and bra?"

   ○ D. "I'd like to see you for a few minutes in your room."

2. Your 35-year-old client says that he never disagrees with anyone and that he has loved everyone he's ever known. What would be your *best* response to this client?

   ○ **A.** "How do you manage to do that?"

   ○ **B.** "That's hard to believe. Most people couldn't do that."

   ○ **C.** "What do you do with feelings of anger or dissatisfaction?"

   ○ **D.** "How did you come to adopt such a way of life?"

3. Your 40-year-old client, who is about to be discharged, says, "I'll bet you hated to graduate." What would be your *best* response to this client?

   ○ **A.** "What prompts you to say that?"

   ○ **B.** "I really enjoyed my graduation."

   ○ **C.** "I hated saying good-bye to some of my friends."

   ○ **D.** "Tell me about how you felt when you graduated."

4. Mr. Crain tried to run away from the hospital 2 days ago. As a result, his grounds privileges were revoked for 1 week. Today he asks you to let him go for a short walk on the grounds. What would be your *best* response to Mr. Crain's request?

   ○ **A.** "Although I think it would be good for you to take a walk, your physician has taken away your grounds privileges."

   ○ **B.** "I understand your grounds privileges have been revoked. I'd be glad to do something with you on the unit."

   ○ **C.** "You decided to leave the hospital 2 days ago without permission. We can't allow you to go outside."

   ○ **D.** "You are not allowed outside. It will be at least 5 more days before grounds privileges are restored."

5. You are sitting in the dayroom when a female client begins to take off her clothing. What is the most reasonable inference for you to make?

   ○ **A.** She is hallucinating.

   ○ **B.** She is sexually preoccupied.

   ○ **C.** Her anxiety is at the severe or panic level.

   ○ **D.** The external environment is too stimulating.

6. The female client described above continues to disrobe in the dayroom. Which of the following nursing actions would be the most therapeutic for such a client?

   ○ **A.** Assist the client in redressing; then take her to her room.

   ○ **B.** Ask the client why she is disrobing in a public place.

   ○ **C.** Continue to observe the client's behavior.

   ○ **D.** Clear the dayroom to give the client privacy.

7. You are working with a client who has just stimulated your anger by using a condescending tone of voice with you. Which of the following responses would be the most therapeutic way to acknowledge the effect upon you?

   ○ **A.** "I feel angry when I hear that tone of voice."

   ○ **B.** "You make me so angry when you talk to me that way."

   ○ **C.** "Are you trying to make me angry?"

   ○ **D.** "Why do you do that with me?"

8. George Akin, age 36, has just spent the last 10 minutes complaining about the hospital and his physician; he concludes his monologue by saying, "The nurses around here are insensitive and incompetent." What is your *best* response to Mr. Akin?

   ○ **A.** "It is difficult to be sensitive to a person who complains as you do."

   ○ **B.** "I don't appreciate your verbal abusiveness. We'll talk later when you cool down."

   ○ **C.** "Sometimes the things we cannot tolerate in others are the very things we cannot tolerate in ourselves."

   ○ **D.** "Give me a specific example of a nurse being insensitive or incompetent."

9. Harold Mays, a client on your unit, says that the Mafia has a "contract" out on him. He refuses to leave his semiprivate room and insists on "frisking" his roommate before allowing him to enter. Which of the following actions should you take *first*?

   ○ **A.** Have Mr. Mays transferred to a private room.

   ○ **B.** Acknowledge Mr. Mays's fear when he refuses to leave his room or wants to "frisk" his roommate.

   ○ **C.** Transfer the roommate to another room.

   ○ **D.** Lock Mr. Mays out of his room for a short while each day so that he can see that he is safe.

10. You are working with a young woman who has acute schizophrenia. As you approach her, you notice that she is sitting on her bed in a puddle of urine. She is playing in it, smiling, and softly singing a children's song. Which of the following would be the *best* nursing action to take?

○ **A.** Admonish her for not using the bathroom.

○ **B.** Firmly tell her that her behavior is unacceptable.

○ **C.** Ask her if she is ready to get cleaned up now.

○ **D.** Help her to the shower, and change the bedclothes.

11. Georgia Kim, age 38, has been hospitalized twice previously for episodes of hypomania (bipolar disorder). She talks incessantly in an exhilarated fashion and jumps from one activity to another, showing a limited concentration span. She also intrudes on the activities of others. At one point, Ms. Kim approaches an immobilized, depressed client and enthusiastically invites him to dance. What is the nurse's *best* intervention?

○ **A.** Tell Ms. Kim that her behavior is inappropriate.

○ **B.** Ask the other client how he feels about dancing with Ms. Kim.

○ **C.** Do nothing if the other client appears comfortable.

○ **D.** Take Ms. Kim to a quiet environment, and engage her in a structured activity.

12. Rick Ellis, one of your clients, is suffering from depression. He refuses to go to occupational therapy (OT) because he says it is boring. Which of the following would be the *best* action for you to take?

○ **A.** State firmly that you will escort him to OT.

○ **B.** Arrange with OT for Mr. Ellis to do a project on the unit.

○ **C.** Ask Mr. Ellis to talk about why OT is boring.

○ **D.** Arrange for Mr. Ellis not to attend OT until he feels better.

13. Mary Long, another client with depression, says that she is "no good" and tells you to "spend your time with someone else." Which of the following would be the most therapeutic response to this client?

○ **A.** "I am going to stay with you for the next 15 minutes."

○ **B.** "Since I am assigned to you, I will stay with you."

○ **C.** "Why do you put yourself down like that?"

○ **D.** "What do you mean when you say that you are no good?"

14. Charles Moore, age 42, returns to the hospital at 9:00 p.m. from a city day-pass. He is 3 hours late. The nurse smells alcohol on his breath. His speech is slurred, and his gait is unsteady. Which of the following would be the nurse's *best* response?

- ○ **A.** "Mr. Moore, why are you 3 hours late in returning from your city day-pass?"
- ○ **B.** "Mr. Moore, how much did you drink tonight? You know drinking is against the rules."
- ○ **C.** "Mr. Moore, I am disappointed that you have not been more responsible with your city day-pass."
- ○ **D.** "Mr. Moore, I want you to go to bed now. We'll talk in the morning."

15. Louis Macon, a client on your unit, tells you that his wife's nagging really gets on his nerves. He asks you if you will talk with her about her nagging during their family session tomorrow afternoon. Which of the following would be the most therapeutic response to Mr. Macon?

- ○ **A.** "Tell me more specifically about her complaints."
- ○ **B.** "Can you think why she might nag you so much?"
- ○ **C.** "I'll help you think about how to bring this up yourself tomorrow afternoon."
- ○ **D.** "Why do you want me to initiate this in tomorrow's session rather than you?"

16. One of your new clients is experiencing delusions. Which of the following nursing actions is important when working with a delusional client?

- ○ **A.** Question the client about the delusion.
- ○ **B.** Point out to the client why the delusion is false.
- ○ **C.** Go along with the delusion until the client's anxiety decreases.
- ○ **D.** Refocus the client toward a structured activity.

17. Donna Jones, age 32, is admitted to the psychiatric unit after experiencing a conversion reaction. The nurse initially establishes short- and long-term goals. Which of the following is a long-term goal?

- ○ **A.** The client will verbalize her feelings and anxiety.
- ○ **B.** The client will participate in unit activities.
- ○ **C.** The client will gain insight into her paralysis.
- ○ **D.** The client will perform self-care.

18. During the working phase of the nurse-client relationship, Donna says to her primary nurse, "You think I could walk if I wanted to, don't you?" Which of the following would be the nurse's *best* response?

○ **A.** "Yes, if you really wanted to, you could."

○ **B.** "Tell me why you're concerned about what I think."

○ **C.** "Do you think you could walk if you wanted to?"

○ **D.** "I think you are unable to walk now, whatever the cause."

19. Because of an illness in your extended family, you missed your last appointment with Ms. Hardy, a client on a psychiatric unit. As you enter the unit today, Ms. Hardy rushes toward you and says in a loud and pressured tone of voice, "I can't help you." Which of the following would be the *best* response to make?

○ **A.** "Who told you why I wasn't here last time?"

○ **B.** "How do you feel about my missing our last meeting?"

○ **C.** "I'm not sure what you mean when you say you can't help me."

○ **D.** "Thank you for your concern about my being absent."

20. A young female client who is in a psychiatric facility stiffly walks up to the nurse and says in a flat tone of voice, "I'm dead. The staff just killed me." Which of the following would be the *most* therapeutic response?

○ **A.** "What did the staff do to kill you?"

○ **B.** "You look like you're alive to me."

○ **C.** "Would you like to lie down for a while?"

○ **D.** "I'm not sure what you mean."

21. Mrs. Lori Saunders reports to her therapy group that she has begun to practice a conscious relaxation technique. She is pleased with its effectiveness in reducing her need to wash her hands. One member responds by saying that conscious relaxation is a bunch of nonsense. A nurse is serving as group leader. Which of the following would be the *best* intervention for the nurse to make at this point?

○ **A.** Smile and change the focus of discussion.

○ **B.** Ask the group member why he thinks the technique worked so well for Mrs. Saunders.

○ **C.** Foster group cohesiveness by asking the member to keep negative opinions to himself.

○ **D.** Ask the member to share his understanding of and experience with conscious relaxation.

22. Jeremy Jenkins, a client on the psychiatric unit, has obtained a Sunday pass to go to a family reunion picnic. He is currently taking fluphenazine (Prolixin). Which of the following instructions should the nurse give to Mr. Jenkins?

○ **A.** Wear plenty of sunscreen at the picnic.

○ **B.** Drink an extra quart of fluid at the picnic.

○ **C.** Avoid eating cheese at the picnic.

○ **D.** Engage in picnic activities only in a limited manner.

23. Mr. Robert Werk, age 47, is suffering from acute exogenous depression that developed after his wife's death. He is taking Nardil, a monoamine oxidase (MAO) inhibitor, to control symptoms of the depression. Other than his current problem, he has no history of mental or physical illness. He has been admitted to the hospital with a marked blood pressure elevation. Your initial assessment would include a thorough neurologic evaluation. What is the rationale for such an evaluation?

○ **A.** Acute exogenous depression is characterized by enhanced platelet activity and cerebrovascular accidents.

○ **B.** Acute exogenous depression, when treated with a MAO inhibitor, can result in permanent neurologic impairment if therapeutic dosages are exceeded.

○ **C.** MAO inhibitors are associated with acute hypertensive crisis related to the intake of certain foods and drugs.

○ **D.** Blood pressure elevation may signal the onset of the depression's manic phase.

24. Mrs. Mae Bowman has been on your nursing unit for 1 week. Her nighttime confusion and wandering have decreased but continue to occur at least once each night. During a team meeting, a staff member recommends that Mrs. Bowman be placed in restraints at night. Which of the following would be your *best* response?

○ **A.** "Restraints are used only to protect the health and safety of clients."

○ **B.** "Restraints may be used for purposes of discipline."

○ **C.** "Restraints may be used to control a client's verbal outbursts."

○ **D.** "Restraints are effective in reducing the number of client falls."

25. Bill Johnson, age 19, just arrived on your psychiatric unit from the emergency department. Unemployed, he has been living at home with his parents. His diagnosis is personality disorder, and he exhibits manipulative behavior. You go over the unit rules with him. Mr. Johnson asks, "Can I go to the snack shop just one time, and then I will answer whatever questions you have?" Which of the following would be your *best* response to this client?

○ **A.** "Okay, but hurry up. I need to finish your assessment."

○ **B.** "Okay, but only for 5 minutes."

○ **C.** "No, you can't go."

○ **D.** "No, you can't go. The rules here are for everyone."

26. Lisa Roda, age 22, has been diagnosed with antisocial personality disorder. She has been having problems since age 15 when she ran away from home. Lisa has had two broken marriages and cannot keep a job for more than 2 months. She has had difficulties with the law because of drug abuse and writing bad checks. She has just broken another unit rule, and her phone privileges have been revoked. Lisa states to the nurse, "Can't I just make one more phone call?" Which of the following would be the nurse's *best* response?

○ **A.** "Okay, but don't talk too long."

○ **B.** "Okay, if you promise to obey the rules the rest of the day."

○ **C.** "No, you can't. The rules apply equally to everyone and you broke them."

○ **D.** "No, you can't. Go watch television."

27. Joy and Cynthia are two of six clients who have been attending your group therapy sessions. Before the next session is about to start, Joy tells you that Cynthia has been discussing group business with individuals who are not in the group. Joy is no longer willing to share anything in the group because of Cynthia's "big mouth." Which of the following would be your *best* response to Joy?

○ **A.** "I want you to tell Cynthia what you've just told me."

○ **B.** "How do you know that Cynthia has discussed group business with others?"

○ **C.** "I would also be hesitant about sharing anything else in the group."

○ **D.** "How do you feel about what Cynthia did?"

28. Suzie Marks, age 8, has not gone to school for 3 weeks. Each morning she says she feels sick and has refused to get out of bed. Suzie's mother brings

her to the mental health clinic. Which of the following is *most* important during your first interview with Suzie's mother?

○ **A.** Reassure her that this is probably a phase that Suzie will soon pass through.

○ **B.** Ask her to identify tensions in the home that could be precipitating Suzie's behavior.

○ **C.** Ask her to describe any changes that occurred before Suzie's symptoms developed.

○ **D.** Have her describe each family member's relationship with Suzie.

29. Which of the following would be appropriate during your first interview with Suzie?

○ **A.** Ask her why she doesn't like school anymore.

○ **B.** Have her describe how things were for her right before she started not wanting to go to school anymore.

○ **C.** Tell her that it is okay for her to be afraid to go to school, but that she will have to start going back.

○ **D.** Reassure her that even though things may not be right in her life just now, they soon will be.

30. A nurse is the leader of an inpatient therapy group. One group member accuses the nurse of being far too "pushy" and says the nurse does not have the right to pressure anyone in the group. Which of the following responses would be *most* likely to help the client remain nondefensive?

○ **A.** "I'm sensing that you are uncomfortable in the group."

○ **B.** "Why are you feeling pressured and pushed by me?"

○ **C.** "Can you tell me exactly what it is that is bothering you?"

○ **D.** "Tell me about one time when you felt pushed or pressured."

31. You are working on an eating-disorders hotline. A 27-year-old woman calls in, crying; she says that she feels miserable about her disgusting habit of binging and vomiting. She asks if you can help her. Which of the following would be your *best* response?

○ **A.** "You did the right thing by calling the hotline. We can help you."

○ **B.** "Tell me about your binging and vomiting. Talking about it will help you."

○ **C.** "Let me give you the name and number of a good therapist. Will you call him?"

○ **D.** "I'm a nurse, and I want you to come to our clinic immediately. I will be waiting for you."

32. Mrs. Ann Pepper, age 59, has been diagnosed with Alzheimer's disease. She has been wearing the same dirty and torn undergarments for several days. The nurse contacts her daughters and asks them to bring in other clothing. Which of the following interventions would *best* prevent further regression in Mrs. Pepper's personal hygiene habits?

○ **A.** Encourage Mrs. Pepper to perform as much self-care as she can.

○ **B.** Make Mrs. Pepper assume responsibility for her physical care.

○ **C.** Assign a staff member to take over Mrs. Pepper's physical care.

○ **D.** Accept Mrs. Pepper's need to go without bathing and to wear dirty clothing if she so desires.

33. Mrs. Pepper becomes verbally and physically abusive when the nurse enters her room to assist with her daily care. Which of the following interventions should the nurse engage in *first*?

○ **A.** Check orders for physical and chemical restraints.

○ **B.** Set firm limits verbally.

○ **C.** Give clear directions while gently securing the client's arms to prevent her from hitting the nurse.

○ **D.** Leave the room and let the angry, hostile behavior work itself out.

34. Jackie Spiro, a 28-year-old accountant, is admitted to the neurologic unit after a sudden onset of blindness the day before an important project is due for her boss. Preliminary evaluation and testing reveal no positive findings. The physician's initial reaction is that Jackie may be demonstrating a defense mechanism. Which of the following defense mechanisms might Jackie be using?

○ **A.** Repression

○ **B.** Transference

○ **C.** Reaction formation

○ **D.** Conversion

35. Carol Benz, age 40, is brought to the hospital by her husband because she has refused to get out of bed for 2 days. She will not eat, has been neglecting her household responsibilities, and is tired all of the time. Her diagnosis on admission is major depression. Carol is being interviewed by the admitting nurse. Which of the following questions would be *most* appropriate for the nurse to ask at this time?

○ **A.** "What has been troubling you?"

○ **B.** "Why do you dislike yourself, Carol?"

○ **C.** "How do you feel about your life?"

○ **D.** "What can we do to help?"

36. Carol begins to improve and participates in treatment programs on the unit. You recognize that Carol is ready for discharge when she:

○ **A.** Asks the staff for advice about how to handle her future.

○ **B.** Speaks to her employer about returning to work.

○ **C.** Identifies her weaknesses and plans to work on them.

○ **D.** Discusses her plan to return home and continue outpatient treatment.

37. An abused child is expected to stay on your unit for 3 to 4 weeks. Which of the following would be the *best* nursing assignment for this client?

○ **A.** A different primary nurse each day

○ **B.** A primary nurse who is transferring next week to another unit

○ **C.** The same primary nurse each day

○ **D.** A new primary nurse every 3 days

38. Heather Rankin, a 24-year-old secretary, is transferred to your psychiatric unit. Her husband says that she has been overeating and that she vomits soon after she eats. Her weight stays about the same. Which of the following medical diagnoses would apply in this case?

○ **A.** Anorexia nervosa

○ **B.** Bulimia

○ **C.** Bulimarexia

○ **D.** Dysthymia

39. Janet Bower, a 45-year-old housewife, has been treated for major depression for the past 15 years. She reports to her physician that she has been experiencing complications from her usual antidepressant, so the physician prescribes a monoamine oxidase (MAO) inhibitor instead. Which of the following foods should Janet be instructed to avoid once she begins taking the MAO inhibitor?

○ **A.** Smoked salmon

○ **B.** Milk and egg products

○ **C.** Honey

○ **D.** Dried nuts

40. After teaching Janet about the adverse effects associated with certain foods and MAO inhibitors, you begin to caution her about possible interactions between MAOs and other drugs. Which of the following drugs should Janet avoid while taking an MAO inhibitor?

○ **A.** Aspirin

○ **B.** Anticoagulants

○ **C.** Antihistamines

○ **D.** Antihypertensives

41. Mrs. Ronda Scarsen, age 72, frequently wanders away from home and is unable to provide directions on how to return. Which of the following is the *best* instruction to Mrs. Scarsen's daughter on how to ensure her safety?

○ **A.** "Your mother's condition is temporary; it will soon pass."

○ **B.** "If I were you, I would move in with your mother."

○ **C.** "It's best that you have your mother committed."

○ **D.** "It's important that someone is available at all times for your mother's safety."

42. Charlene Davis, age 15, was admitted to the eating disorders unit 2 days ago. She is 5′ 6″ tall and weighs 92 lb. You are her primary nurse and will be having your first one-on-one session with Charlene today. Which of the following represents the *most* important information that you should gather from Charlene during this first session?

○ **A.** A detailed history of her eating habits

○ **B.** How she views her current situation

○ **C.** What she expects to achieve during hospitalization

○ **D.** How she views herself in relation to her peers

43. Since being admitted to the eating disorders unit, Charlene has dropped from 92 lb to 89 lb. Which of the following would be the *best* nursing action at this point?

○ **A.** Place Charlene on a behavior modification program.

○ **B.** Place Charlene on bed rest until she regains the 3 lb.

○ **C.** Tell Charlene that you are concerned about the 3-lb loss.

○ **D.** Ask Charlene which foods she would feel most comfortable eating.

44. Charlene's weight increases to 93 lb. Which of the following would be the *best* nursing action to take now?

○ **A.** Suggest that Charlene be discharged and treated on an outpatient basis.

○ **B.** Set weekly treatment goals for Charlene to review in group therapy.

○ **C.** Negotiate with Charlene about the continuing terms of the treatment plan.

○ **D.** Engage in weekly psychotherapy sessions with Charlene and her family.

45. A very shy, retiring client hands you several capsules he found "on the floor." Several clients are receiving this particular medication. Which of the following actions should you take *first*?

○ **A.** Restrict all clients' privileges until you find out what is happening.

○ **B.** Initiate a unit-wide search to determine whether any more drugs can be found.

○ **C.** Observe all clients carefully during and after they receive the medication in question.

○ **D.** Call all the clients together, and ask if anyone knows how these capsules got on the floor.

46. One of your clients tells you that nothing good has ever happened to her. You use a cognitive approach in your work with clients. Which of the following responses represents the cognitive approach?

○ **A.** "You must feel terrible."

○ **B.** "How have you come to that conclusion?"

○ **C.** "Hasn't your relationship with me been good?"

○ **D.** "How does that make you feel?"

47. Frank Shaffer asks you if it's okay for him to leave your one-on-one session to get a drink of water. One of Mr. Shaffer's treatment goals is to promote personal growth. Which of the following would be the *best* response to Mr. Shaffer's question?

○ **A.** "Whether or not you get a drink is your decision."

○ **B.** "Your leaving to get a drink would be disruptive."

○ **C.** "We're almost finished; do you think you can wait?"

○ **D.** "You should have taken care of that before we started."

48. Your client's mother died unexpectedly about 8 months ago. The client still has many regrets about not coming to closure with her mother over two specific issues. You plan to use a Gestalt approach when working with the client. Which of the following interventions represents the Gestalt approach?

○ **A.** Changing the ego state from which the client operates

○ **B.** Teaching the client about the stages of grieving

○ **C.** Identifying the thoughts leading to the client's distress

○ **D.** Having the client "talk" to her mother

49. Judd Roberts, age 24, is an intrusive client, constantly invading the physical and social spaces of staff and peers. He does not comprehend that his behavior is inappropriate. Which of the following descriptions represents the Sullivanian theory?

○ **A.** Judd experiences severe-level anxiety.

○ **B.** Judd operates in the prototaxic mode.

○ **C.** Judd exhibits problems with intimacy versus isolation.

○ **D.** Judd has an ineffective ego and overactive id.

50. Mrs. Miller is admitted to the oncology unit for treatment of uterine cancer. Routine laboratory tests reveal a total white blood cell count below normal limits, with a marked reduction in the neutrophil count. Her physician orders lithium carbonate, 300 mg t.i.d. by mouth. When the drug is administered for the first time, her husband becomes angry and follows you out into the hallway. He whispers loudly, "That drug is for crazy people. My wife has cancer!" Which of the following is your *best* response to Mr. Miller?

○ **A.** "We understand your wife has cancer, Mr. Miller. This drug is being given for other purposes."

○ **B.** "Calm down, Mr. Miller. Would you like to talk about it?"

○ **C.** "You are angry because you think we don't know what's wrong with your wife?"

○ **D.** "I'm sorry you are upset, Mr. Miller. Let me explain why the physician ordered lithium."

51. Mrs. Miller has been receiving lithium for 2 weeks. She also has been receiving a number of chemotherapeutic drugs that cause her to feel nauseated and anorexic, making it difficult to distinguish the early signs of lithium toxicity. Which of the following signs would indicate lithium toxicity at serum drug levels below 1.5 mEq/liter?

○ **A.** Hyperpyrexia

○ **B.** Marked analgesia and lethargy

○ **C.** Hypotonic reflexes, with muscle weakness

○ **D.** Renal failure

52. David Reese is a client on an inpatient psychiatric unit at a community mental health center. He has a history of aggression. One of the nurses observes Mr. Reese pacing continually up and down the hallway. Which of the following would be the nurse's *best* response?

    ○ A. "If you can't relax, you could go to your room."

    ○ B. "Would you like your antianxiety medication now?"

    ○ C. "You're pacing, Mr. Reese. What's going on?"

    ○ D. "Let's go play a game of pool, Mr. Reese."

53. A voluntarily admitted client asks to be discharged from the hospital against medical advice. Which of the following *must* the nurse assess before the client is discharged?

    ○ A. Ability to care for self

    ○ B. Danger to self and others

    ○ C. Level of psychosis

    ○ D. Intended compliance with treatment after discharge

54. Marie Sullivan, a 24-year-old schizophrenic, is admitted to the unit in a catatonic state. The physician prescribes haloperidol (Haldol) 5 mg t.i.d. Four days after admission, Marie comes out of the coma and gradually begins to take care of herself. She says that the FBI is after her because she was a key figure in the Iran-Contra affair with Oliver North. Which of the following would be the nurse's *best* response?

    ○ A. "How long have you known Oliver North?"

    ○ B. "You are Marie and you do not know Oliver North."

    ○ C. "Why do you think the FBI would be looking for you here?"

    ○ D. "You must feel important. Can I accompany you to breakfast?"

55. Carl Allen, a 45-year-old accountant, has been admitted to the hospital because of extreme agitation. He feels that he must pace the floor a specific number of times each day or "something terrible" will happen to him. He has engaged in this behavior most of his adult life. Which of the following would be the *most* appropriate response for the nurse to make?

    ○ A. "Mr. Allen, nothing will happen to you. You must stop this behavior."

    ○ B. "Mr. Allen, are you looking for attention? There are other ways you can get this attention."

    ○ C. "Mr. Allen, this behavior has created some difficulty for you. It might help if we talked about why you find it necessary to do this."

    ○ D. "I understand your need to work off excess energy."

56. Nelson Della, age 39, is suffering from depression. He says, "I'm a failure. I can't even cope with little things anymore." Which of the following would be the *most* appropriate nursing response?

    ○ **A.** "Do you feel like you don't deserve to feel good about yourself?"

    ○ **B.** "I know you feel like that now, but you'll feel differently when you get better."

    ○ **C.** "What has happened to make you feel like such a failure?"

    ○ **D.** "It sounds as if you are feeling pretty overwhelmed right now."

57. Lillian Hammond comes into the emergency services department of the community mental health center. She pleads with the nurse, "Make my husband stop drinking." Which of the following would be the nurse's *best* response?

    ○ **A.** "Tell me exactly why you are so concerned about your husband's drinking."

    ○ **B.** "I can't do anything about your husband's drinking unless he comes here for help."

    ○ **C.** "I can see you are feeling distraught. Tell me exactly what made you come here today."

    ○ **D.** "I can see you are feeling distraught. It's hard to live with someone who abuses alcohol."

58. You have been working with a client who has an anxiety disorder. During one of your meetings, the client abruptly says, "I really love you." Which of the following would be your *best* response?

    ○ **A.** "Why do you think you love me?"

    ○ **B.** "What do you mean you love me? Are you sure?"

    ○ **C.** "I can sense you have strong feelings about me. Let's talk about that."

    ○ **D.** "It's nice to share feelings with others. What other feelings could we share?"

59. A 15-year-old client with anorexia nervosa asks you if she has done any permanent damage to her body. Which of the following would be the *most* therapeutic reply?

    ○ **A.** "It's too early to determine that yet."

    ○ **B.** "Have you asked your physician that question?"

    ○ **C.** "What has prompted you to ask that question?"

    ○ **D.** "Did someone say you have damaged your body?"

60. Tom Scalia, an acutely manic client, kisses you on the lips and asks you to marry him. You are taken by surprise. How should you respond?

○ **A.** Seclude him for his inappropriate behavior.

○ **B.** Ask him what he's trying to prove by his behavior.

○ **C.** Have him help you fold some laundry.

○ **D.** Tell him that you find his behavior offensive.

Answers and rationales

The question number appears in boldface type, followed by the letter of the correct answer. The text then provides rationales for correct answers and, where appropriate, for incorrect options. To help you evaluate your knowledge base and application of nursing behaviors, each question has been classified as follows:

NP = Phase of the nursing process

CN = Client need

CL = Cognitive level.

1. Answer: D

Requesting a private conversation demonstrates respect for the client while removing her from an embarrassing situation. Option A is incorrect because the client would have worn more clothing if she had thought that she needed it, and, because her anxiety level is severe, she cannot independently follow through with instructions. Options B and C are incorrect because they are insensitive to the social context in which the client's behavior is occurring.

NP: Implementation

CN: Psychosocial integrity

CL: Synthesis

2. Answer: D

Inquiring about the client's way of life allows for further exploration of the message he is trying to convey. Option A has too narrow a focus and does not permit maximal exploration of the client's experience. Option B is incorrect because the client could misinterpret it as a challenge and become even more defensive than he already is. Option C is incorrect because the nurse should not identify the client's feelings for him.

NP: Assessment

CN: Psychosocial integrity

CL: Synthesis

3. Answer: A

Asking the client to reveal what prompted his remark allows for further exploration of his statement. Options B and C serve as blocks to such exploration, improperly focusing on the nurse's feelings rather than the client's. Option D is too concrete a response and misses the point.

NP: Intervention

CN: Psychosocial integrity

CL: Synthesis

4. Answer: B

This response restates the imposed limitation without demeaning the client and also conveys the nurse's willingness to spend time with the client. Option A is incorrect because the nurse, in assigning sole responsibility for the revocation to the physician, would be engaging in staff splitting. Option C implies that the staff is unable to make decisions; use of the word "can't" implies helplessness. Although Option D adequately restates the imposed limitation, it gives no indication of the nurse's willingness to spend time with the client.

NP: Intervention

CN: Psychosocial integrity

CL: Synthesis

5. Answer: C

Clients with mild or moderate anxiety do not behave in socially inappropriate ways, so this client's anxiety must be at the severe or panic level. Options A, B, and D are all incorrect because the clinical situation does not include sufficient data to support these inferences.

NP: Assessment

CN: Psychosocial integrity

CL: Application

6. Answer: A

The most therapeutic nursing action would be to help the client get dressed and then take her to her room. The nurse should not permit the client to do anything in public that will embarrass the client later. Option B is incorrect because the client's anxiety level does not permit her to solve problems independently. Option C is incorrect because the client's anxiety is high enough that she will continue her behavior and further embarrass herself. Option D does not set appropriate limits on her socially inappropriate behavior.

NP: Intervention

CN: Psychosocial integrity

CL: Application

7. Answer: A

This response (known as an "I" message, as opposed to a "you" message) allows you to provide feedback without making the client responsible for your reaction. Option B is accusatory and blocks communication. Option C is a challenging remark that can lead to power struggles, lower the client's self-esteem, and block opportunities for open communication. Option D is incorrect because "Why" questions put the client on the defensive.

NP: Implementation

CN: Psychosocial integrity

CL: Synthesis

8. Answer: D

Asking the client to support his contention with a concrete example compels him to specify events and may enhance his ability to view the situation more objectively. Option A may only serve to exacerbate the client's already negative behavior. Option B halts the conversation, thereby blocking therapeutic communication. Option C is too confrontational.

NP: Assessment

CN: Psychosocial integrity

CL: Synthesis

9. Answer: B

Acknowledging underlying feelings may help defuse the client's anxiety without promoting his delusional thinking. This, in turn, may help the client distinguish between his emotional state and external reality. Options A and C are not the preferred actions because transferring either client to another room would validate the client's delusional thinking. (If Option B does not work, however, then Option C would be the next best action, to protect the roommate and to control Mr. Mays's anxiety.) Option D — locking the client out of his room — would probably further escalate his anxiety and stimulate aggressive acting-out behavior; it also would deprive him of a place where he can feel safe.

NP: Implementation

CN: Psychosocial integrity

CL: Synthesis

10. Answer: D

The client has panic-level anxiety. You must help her meet self-care needs. Options A, B, and C would be inappropriate for a client with panic anxiety; she could not "hear" you, and she would require much more structure and assistance than those options afford.

NP: Implementation

CN: Psychosocial integrity

CL: Application

11. Answer: D

Because Ms. Kim cannot set limits on her own behavior, the nurse must do so. Structured activities tend to benefit clients with bipolar disorder, who typically need assistance in appropriately channeling their energy. Option A insufficiently addresses the client's severe anxiety level. Option B not only puts the other client in an awkward position but also condones Ms. Kim's inappropriate behavior. Option C fails to address the inappropriate behavior, which, if left unchecked, will eventually create anxiety in others who are in her immediate environment.

NP: Implementation

CN: Safe, effective care environment

CL: Application

12. Answer: A

If given the chance, a depressed client typically elects to remain immobilized. You must insist that the client participate in occupational therapy (OT). Option B validates and reinforces the client's desire to avoid going to OT. Option C addresses an invalid issue (most things bore depressed persons) while avoiding the real issue (the client's need for therapy). Option D incorrectly suggests that the client isn't capable of participating in OT, further undermining an already lowered self-esteem.

NP: Implementation

CN: Psychosocial integrity

CL: Application

13. Answer: A

This response conveys your interest in the client while communicating firmly that you will not be pushed away. Option B suggests that staying with the client is a duty you are performing unwillingly, which may further diminish her already low self-esteem. Options C and D inappropriately focus on the negative by inviting the client to expand on the reasons why she is no good, further reinforcing her negative self-image.

NP: Implementation

CN: Psychosocial integrity

CL: Application

14. Answer: D

The client can best process his behavior when he is no longer under the influence of alcohol. Option A is incorrect because the client (who is intoxicated and who may be experiencing a blackout) may invent excuses for his whereabouts. Option B is incorrect because any consumption of alcohol by the client is unacceptable; the amount is irrelevant. Option C is inappropriate because the nurse's statement is judgmental.

NP: Implementation

CN: Psychosocial integrity

CL: Application

15. Answer: C

The client needs to learn how to communicate directly with his wife about her behavior. Your assistance will enable him to practice a new skill and will communicate your confidence in his ability to confront this situation directly. Options A and B inappropriately direct attention away from the client and toward his wife, who is not present. Option D implies that there might be a legitimate reason for you to assume responsibility for something that rightfully belongs to Mr. Macon. Instead of focusing on his problems, he will waste precious time convincing you why you should do his work.

NP: Analysis

CN: Psychosocial integrity

CL: Analysis

16. Answer: D

Refocusing the client toward a structured activity reinforces reality. Options A and C are incorrect because the nurse should not make delusions seem real. Option B is futile; the more the nurse tries to disprove the delusion, the more the client will cling to it.

NP: Implementation

CN: Psychosocial integrity

CL: Application

17. Answer: C

Having the client gain insight into her paralysis is the only long-term goal listed. Options A, B, and D are short-term goals.

NP: Planning

CN: Psychosocial integrity

CL: Application

18. Answer: D

This response answers the question honestly and nonjudgmentally and helps to preserve the client's self-esteem. Option A is an open and candid response, but it tends to diminish the client's self-esteem. Option B does not answer the client's question and is not helpful. Option C would increase the client's anxiety because her inability to walk is directly related to an unconscious psychological conflict that has not yet been resolved.

NP: Implementation

CN: Psychosocial integrity

CL: Application

19. Answer: C

This response seeks clarification about what Ms. Hardy thinks or feels she should be doing for the nurse; it also allows for exploration of possible feelings of helplessness or uselessness in past situations. Options A, B, and D do not address Ms. Hardy's comment that she cannot help the nurse. Option D also blocks further exploration of the client's feelings.

NP: Implementation

CN: Psychosocial integrity

CL: Application

20. Answer: D

This response seeks further clarification of the client's comment. Option A inappropriately validates the client's misperception. Option B denies the client's experience. Option C ignores the client's statement.

NP: Implementation

CN: Psychosocial integrity

CL: Application

21. Answer: D

This response seeks first to clarify the group member's experience and then to provide an opportunity for the group leader or another member to explain the purpose of conscious relaxation. Option A ignores the issue being discussed. Option B takes the focus away from the client's concern. Option C does not foster group cohesiveness; negative opinions are valid and should not be suppressed.

NP: Implementation

CN: Psychosocial integrity

CL: Application

22. Answer: A

Fluphenazine, an antipsychotic drug, can cause photosensitivity and severe sunburn. Options B and C are incorrect because they do not influence the effects of antipsychotic drugs. Option D is incorrect because antipsychotic drugs do not affect one's ability to engage in usual picnic activities.

NP: Implementation

CL: Health promotion and maintenance

CL: Analysis

23. Answer: C

In combination with monoamine oxidase (MAO) inhibitors, tyramine (a substance found in certain foods and drugs) can cause an acute hypertensive crisis. Option A is incorrect because MAO inhibitors have no effect on platelet activity. Option B is incorrect because MAO inhibitors affect the storage of neurohormones; they have no direct effect on nerve cells and no permanent effect on the body. Option D is incorrect because persons with exogenous depression are not prone to manic episodes.

NP: Assessment

CN: Physiologic integrity

CL: Application

24. Answer: A

Existing laws stipulate the acceptable practices involved in the use of restraints. Protecting the health and safety of the client is the primary reason to use restraints. Options B and C are incorrect because the laws expressly prohibit the use of restraints to control or discipline a client. Option D is incorrect in light of recent research showing that restraints do not significantly reduce client falls.

NP: Planning

CN: Safe, effective care environment

CL: Application

25. Answer: D

This response sets appropriate limits. Options A and B give in to the client's manipulative behavior. Option C does not provide an explanation for the refusal.

NP: Assessment

CN: Psychosocial integrity

CL: Analysis

26. Answer: C

This response enforces the unit rules and explains why the client is not permitted to use the phone. Options A and B do not encourage the client to follow rules. Option D does not explain why the client's request has been refused.

NP: Implementation

CN: Psychosocial integrity

CL: Analysis

27. Answer: A

This response forces Joy to validate her perception directly with Cynthia. Adult behavior includes learning how to be assertive without being hostile. Options B, C, and D do not assist the client in learning this task.

NP: Implementation

CN: Psychosocial integrity

CL: Synthesis

28. Answer: C

This response allows you to assess what could have precipitated Suzie's change in behavior. Option A is incorrect because it provides false reassurance. Option B is incorrect because it makes an assumption without gathering the necessary data. Option D would yield helpful information but not the most important information needed.

NP: Assessment

CN: Psychosocial integrity

CL: Application

29. Answer: B

You need to assess what precipitated Suzie's anxious behavior. Option A is incorrect because Suzie may not be able to answer this question. Option C is an inappropriate comment to make in the initial interview. Option D offers the client false reassurance.

NP: Assessment

CN: Psychosocial integrity

CL: Application

30. Answer: D

This response compels the client to provide a specific example, which may help the client to view the situation more objectively. Option A may be too threatening to the client. Option B could lead to denial if the client feels directly threatened. Option C is inappropriate; if the client knew what was bothering him, he would act differently.

NP: Implementation

CN: Psychosocial integrity

CL: Application

31. Answer: D

This response conveys immediate interest and concern; it tells the caller that you are willing to get involved and provide tangible assistance. Option A does not prompt the caller to take action. Option B is incorrect because talking about the problem won't solve it. Option C is a brush-off, and the caller may hesitate to call someone else.

NP: Implementation

CN: Psychosocial integrity

CL: Analysis

32. Answer: A

This response increases the client's orientation and provides a safe environment while establishing a nurse-client relationship based on trust. Clients with organic mental syndromes tend to fluctuate frequently in terms of their capabilities. Option B would be difficult to accomplish because of the client's confusion. Options C and D diminish the client's independence and self-esteem. Option D also ignores the client's hygiene and grooming needs.

NP: Implementation

CN: Safe, effective care environment

CL: Analysis

33. Answer: B

Clear limits protect the client, staff, and others, and a verbally and physically abusive client sometimes responds to verbal controls. Option A (using restraints to reduce anxiety and control behavior) would be considered only as a last resort, if at all. Option C invades the client's personal space, which might escalate unacceptable behavior. Option D invites the possibility of injury if the client strikes out at the nurse or an imagined threat.

NP: Implementation

CN: Safe, effective care environment

CL: Analysis

34. Answer: D

When feelings become unbearable, the client may rechannel them into physical symptoms. Conversion is a defense mechanism that usually appears shortly after a traumatic or conflict-producing event. The symptoms have no organic cause and often provide attention or an excuse. Repression (Option A) is a defense mechanism by which a person unconsciously keeps unwanted feelings from entering awareness. Transference (Option B) is a defense mechanism by which a person projects feelings, thoughts, and wishes onto others; it can be positive or negative. Reaction formation (Option C) is a defense mechanism by which a person alleviates unresolved emotional conflicts by reinforcing one feeling or impulse and repressing another, thereby disguising the true feelings from the self.

NP: Assessment

CN: Psychosocial integrity

CL: Analysis

35. Answer: C

The nurse must develop nursing interventions based on the client's perceived problems and feelings. Option A asks the client to draw a conclusion, which may be difficult for her to do at this time. Option B asks a "why" question, which can place the client in a defensive position. Option D requires the client to find possible solutions, which is beyond the scope of her present abilities.

NP: Implementation

CN: Psychosocial integrity

CL: Analysis

36. Answer: D

Carol's plan to return home and continue outpatient treatment indicates that she is willing to assume responsibility for her health. Option A implies an unwillingness to accept responsibility. Option B is a positive step, but it will not help the client comprehensively. Option C involves short-term steps taken well before discharge.

NP: Planning

CN: Health promotion and maintenance

CL: Application

37. Answer: C

Assigning the same primary nurse every day will provide continuity of care and will facilitate the development of trust in the nurse-client relationship. Options A, B, and D are not in the best interest of the client, and they will not promote a trusting relationship.

NP: Planning

CN: Psychosocial integrity

CL: Application

38. Answer: B

The client exhibits binging and purging, common signs of bulimia. Option A is incorrect because the client has not experienced weight loss, a common sign of anorexia nervosa. With bulimarexia (Option C), one would expect to see symptoms of both anorexia nervosa and bulimia. Dysthymia (Option D) is a type of depression.

NP: Assessment

CN: Physiologic integrity

CL: Analysis

39. Answer: A

Smoked salmon contains tyramine, a substance that can produce a hypertensive crisis if ingested in a large enough amount. The foods listed in the other options do not contain tyramine.

NP: Planning

CN: Safe, effective care environment

CL: Recognition

40. Answer: D

Hypotension is an adverse effect of MAO inhibitors. Combining an antihypertensive medication with a MAO inhibitor could lead to heart failure. Options A, B, C would not produce a drug-drug interaction.

NP: Planning

CN: Health promotion and maintenance

CL: Analysis

41. Answer: D

This response specifies the conditions necessary for Mrs. Scarsen to be safe while allowing the daughter to determine how she wishes to implement the plan. Option A gives false information. Options B and C impose personal values on the client's daughter.

NP: Implementation

CN: Psychosocial integrity

CL: Synthesis

42. Answer: B

The client's view of her situation determines her behaviors. The nurse cannot plan effective care without first understanding this viewpoint. Option A incorrectly focuses on food and eating habits, which are not the real issue; the client's underlying feelings actually precipitated the eating disorder. Option C is premature. The client doesn't know yet what she expects to achieve during hospitalization. She is probably feeling anxious about being "forced" to gain weight, and she may try to "play games" with the nurse. Option D also is premature. The first session between the client and the nurse should be devoted to establishing rapport and defining the nature of their relationship.

NP: Assessment

CN: Psychosocial integrity

CL: Application

43. Answer: B

Bed rest will conserve the client's energy for weight maintenance or gain. Option A is incorrect because the client will not be able to participate effectively in "talk" therapy until she weighs at least 90 lb. The nurse's verbally expressed concern (Option C) will not prevent further weight loss. Option D is inappropriate; the client at this point is feeling out of control and requires much support and assistance.

NP: Implementation

CN: Physiologic integrity

CL: Application

44. Answer: C

Negotiation gives the client some responsibility for her continued treatment. Option A is premature; the client may begin to lose weight again. Option B takes responsibility away from the client. Option D is premature; psychotherapy may be indicated in the future, but it is not the best intervention at this point.

NP: Implementation

CN: Safe, effective care environment

CL: Application

45. Answer: C

Careful observation is called for in this situation because you need to collect more data. Option A is incorrect because all clients should not be punished for the actions of one or two, and clients are not responsible for the behavior of others. A unit-wide search (Option B) is premature at this point. Calling all of the clients together (Option D) is a viable nursing action, but it has two drawbacks: some clients may interpret it as accusatory, and it could alert the client who is hiding the drug to be more careful.

NP: Implementation

CN: Safe, effective care environment

CL: Synthesis

46. Answer: B

The client is using a cognitive distortion that must be examined. Asking the client to explain or clarify her conclusion focuses on the client's thinking, or cognition. Options A and D focus instead on feelings. Option C focuses on the relationship rather than the thoughts behind the client's statement.

NP: Implementation

CN: Psychosocial integrity

CL: Synthesis

47. Answer: A

This response is the only one that promotes personal growth because it makes the client responsible for his own decision. Options B, C, and D place the nurse in a position of power over the client.

NP: Planning

CN: Psychosocial integrity

CL: Application

48. Answer: D

In the Gestalt mode, the client would resolve unfinished business with her mother by "talking" to her. Option A represents a transactional analysis approach. Option B does not allow for self-discovery and is not part of Gestalt theory. Option C is an approach used in cognitive theory.

NP: Implementation

CN: Psychosocial integrity

CL: Application

49. Answer: B

The client has no concept of appropriate boundaries, indicating lack of differentiation, a key term in Sullivan's theory. Option A refers to one of the anxiety levels specified by Peplau. Option C refers to a developmental stage defined by Erikson. Option D reflects a Freudian approach.

NP: Analysis

CN: Psychosocial integrity

CL: Analysis

50. Answer: D

This response acknowledges and accepts Mr. Miller's anger and offers concrete information to clarify the misunderstanding. Options A and B are defensive communications. Option B also may block communication if Mr. Miller responds with "No". Option C is a defensive restatement of the person's communication.

NP: Intervention

CN: Psychosocial integrity

CL: Synthesis

51. Answer: C

Lithium alters sodium transport in nerve and muscle cells, slowing the speed of impulse transmission. Option A is incorrect because lithium has no known effect on body temperature. Option B is incorrect because lithium does not alter the transmission of pain impulses or cause lethargy. Renal failure (Option D) is a late sign of severe lithium toxicity.

NP: Assessment

CN: Physiologic integrity

CL: Application

52. Answer: C

This response attempts to explore Mr. Reese's feelings. Options A and B assume that the client is anxious (the nurse may be projecting feelings because of the client's history of aggression). Option D ignores what might be going on with Mr. Reese.

NP: Implementation

CN: Safe, effective care environment

CL: Analysis

53. Answer: B

Although each option is an important area for assessment, a voluntary client should not be permitted to leave the hospital if dangerous to self or others.

NP: Assessment

CN: Safe, effective care environment

CL: Application

54. Answer: D

This response focuses on what may be the underlying need for which the delusion was created, and it redirects the client's attention to the current, reality-based situation. Options A, B, and C do not assist the client in giving up the delusion; in fact, they reinforce it.

NP: Implementation

CN: Psychosocial integrity

CL: Analysis

55. Answer: C

This response provides a structure for reducing the client's anxiety, gaining insight into his behavior, and eventually redirecting his anxiety. Options A, B, and D do not assist the client in gaining insight into his behavior, and they may increase his anxiety.

NP: Implementation

CN: Psychosocial integrity

CL: Application

56. Answer: D

This response acknowledges the client's feelings and conveys the nurse's ability to understand them. Options A and C promote a negative self-image rather than attempting to enhance the client's self-esteem. Option B dismisses the client's current feelings.

NP: Implementation

CN: Psychosocial integrity

CL: Application

57. Answer: C

This response acknowledges the client's behavior and asks the client to provide further information about why she is seeking help. Options A and D do not address the reason why Mrs. Hammond is seeking help. Option B does not respond to the client's plea for help.

NP: Implementation

CN: Psychosocial integrity

CL: Application

58. Answer: C

This response indicates that the client's feelings are okay and that you are comfortable with how he feels. Options A and B imply that the client's feelings are not legitimate. Option D evades the issue and only relieves the nurse's anxiety, not the client's.

NP: Implementation

CN: Psychosocial integrity

CL: Synthesis

59. Answer: C

This response enables you to collect more information from the client. Options A and B cut off the discussion. Option D is too specific and may inhibit the client from elaborating further.

NP: Implementation

CN: Psychosocial integrity

CL: Synthesis

60. Answer: C

Having the client help with laundry rechannels his energy in a positive activity. Option A does not take into account that the client needs direction and structure, not seclusion. Option B ignores the client's impaired judgment and poor impulse control. Option D does not assist the client in controlling the behavior.

NP: Implementation

CN: Psychosocial integrity

CL: Application

Analyzing the post-test

Total the number of *incorrect* responses to the post-test. A score of 1 to 9 indicates that you have an excellent knowledge base and that you are well prepared for the certification examination; a score of 10 to 14 indicates adequate preparation, although more study or improvement in test-taking skills is recommended; a score of 15 or more indicates the need for intensive study before taking the certification examination.

For a more detailed analysis of your performance, complete the self-diagnostic profile worksheet on page 230.

Post-test self-diagnostic profile

In the top row of boxes, record the number of each question you answered incorrectly. Then, beneath each question number, check the box that corresponds to the reason you answered the question incorrectly, along with the category of client need and nursing process for that question. Finally, tabulate the number of check marks on each line in the right-hand column marked "Totals". You now have an individualized profile of weak areas that require further study or improvement in test-taking ability before you take the Psychiatric and Mental Health Nursing Certification Examination.

QUESTION NUMBER																								TOTALS
Test-taking skills																								
1. Misread question																								
2. Missed important point																								
3. Forgot fact or concept																								
4. Applied wrong fact or concept																								
5. Drew wrong conclusion																								
6. Incorrectly evaluated distractors																								
7. Mistakenly filled in wrong circle																								
8. Read into question																								
9. Guessed wrong																								
10. Misunderstood question																								
Client need																								
1. Safe, effective care environment																								
2. Physiologic integrity																								
3. Psychosocial integrity																								
4. Health promotion and maintenance																								
Nursing process																								
1. Assessment																								
2. Analysis																								
3. Planning																								
4. Implementation																								
5. Evaluation																								

Appendix A: Standards of psychiatric and mental health nursing practice

In 1973, the American Nurses Association issued standards to help improve the quality of care provided by psychiatric and mental health nurses. These standards, last revised in 1982, apply to generalists and specialists working in any setting in which psychiatric and mental health nursing is practiced. Standards V-F (psychotherapy) and X (community health systems) apply specifically to the specialist. Listed below are the standards for professional practice and professional performance, along with their rationales.

Professional practice standards

Standard I. Theory

The nurse applies appropriate theory that is scientifically sound as a basis for decisions regarding nursing practice.

Rationale

Psychiatric and mental health nursing is characterized by the application of relevant theories to explain phenomena of concern to nurses and to provide a basis for intervention and subsequent evaluation of that intervention. A primary source of knowledge for practice rests on the scholarly conceptualizations of psychiatric and mental health nursing practice and on research findings generated from interdisciplinary and cross-disciplinary studies of human behavior. The nurse's use of selected theories provides comprehensive, balanced perceptions of clients' characteristics, diagnoses, or presenting conditions.

Standard II. Data Collection

The nurse continuously collects data that are comprehensive, accurate, and systematic.

Rationale

Effective interviewing, behavioral observation, and physical and mental health assessment enable the nurse to reach sound conclusions and plan appropriate interventions with the client.

Standard III. Diagnosis

The nurse utilizes nursing diagnoses and standard classifications of mental disorders to express conclusions supported by recorded assessment data and current scientific premises.

Rationale

Nursing's logical basis for providing care rests on the recognition and identification of those actual or potential health problems that are within the scope of nursing practice.

Standard IV. Planning

The nurse develops a nursing care plan with specific goals and interventions delineating nursing actions unique to each client's needs.

Rationale

The nursing care plan is used to guide therapeutic intervention and effectively achieve the desired outcomes.

Standard V. Intervention

The nurse intervenes, as guided by the nursing care plan, to implement nursing actions that promote, maintain, or restore physical and mental health, prevent illness, and effect rehabilitation.

Rationale

Mental health is one aspect of general health and well-being. Nursing actions reflect an appreciation for the hierarchy of human needs and include interventions for all aspects of physical and mental health and illness.

Standard V-A. Intervention: Psychotherapeutic Interventions

The nurse uses psychotherapeutic interventions to assist clients in regaining or improving their previous coping abilities and to prevent further disability.

Rationale

Individuals with and without mental health problems often respond to health problems in a dysfunctional manner. During counseling, interviewing, crisis or emergency intervention, or daily interaction, nurses diagnose dysfunctional behaviors, engage clients in noting such behaviors, and assist clients in modifying those behaviors.

Standard V-B. Intervention: Health Teaching

The nurse assists clients, families, and groups to achieve satisfying and productive patterns of living through health teaching.

Rationale

Health teaching is an essential part of the nurse's role with those who have mental health problems. Every interaction can be utilized as a teaching-learning situation. Formal and informal teaching methods can be used in working with individuals, families, groups, and the community. Emphasis is on understanding principles of mental health as well as on developing ways of coping with mental health problems. Client adherence to treatment regimens increases when health teaching is an integral part of the client's care.

Standard V-C. Intervention: Activities of Daily Living

The nurse uses the activities of daily living in a goal-directed way to foster adequate self-care and physical and mental well-being of clients.

Rationale

A major portion of one's daily life is spent in some form of activity related to health and well-being. An individual's developmental and intellectual levels, emotional state, and physical limitations may be reflected in these activities. Nurses are the primary professional health care providers who interact with clients on a day-to-day basis around the tasks of daily living. Therefore, the nurse has a unique opportunity to assess and intervene in these processes in order to encourage constructive changes in the client's behavior so that each child, adolescent, and adult can realize his potential for growth and health or maintain that level previously achieved.

Standard V-D. Intervention: Somatic Therapies

The nurse uses knowledge of somatic therapies and applies related clinical skills in working with clients.

Rationale

Various treatment modalities may be needed by clients during the course of illness. Pertinent clinical observations and judgments are made concerning the effect of drugs and other somatic treatments used in the therapeutic program.

Standard V-E. Intervention: Therapeutic Environment

The nurse provides, structures, and maintains a therapeutic environment in collaboration with the client and other health care providers.

Rationale

The nurse works with the client in a variety of environmental settings, such as inpatient, residential, day-care, and home. The environment contributes in positive and negative ways to the client's state of health or illness. When it serves the client's interest as an inherent part of the overall nursing care plan, the setting is structured or altered.

Standard V-F. Intervention: Psychotherapy

The nurse utilizes advanced clinical expertise in individual, group, and family psychotherapy; child psychotherapy; and other treatment modalities to function as a psychotherapist and recognizes professional accountability for nursing practice.

Rationale

Acceptance of the role of psychotherapist entails primary responsibility for the treatment of clients and entrance into a contractual agreement. This contract includes a commitment to see a client through the problem presented or to assist the client in finding other appropriate assistance. It also includes an explicit definition of the relationship, the respective role of each person in the relationship, and what can be realistically expected of each person.

Standard VI. Evaluation

The nurse evaluates client responses to nursing actions in order to revise the data base, nursing diagnoses, and nursing care plan.

Rationale

Nursing care is a dynamic process that implies alterations in data, diagnoses, or plans previously made.

Professional performance standards

Standard VII. Peer Review

The nurse participates in peer review and other means of evaluation to assure quality of nursing care provided for clients.

Rationale

Evaluation of the quality of nursing care through examination of the clinical practice of nurses is one way to fulfill the profession's obligation to ensure that consumers are provided excellence in care. Peer review and other quality assurance procedures are utilized in this endeavor.

Standard VIII. Continuing Education

The nurse assumes responsibility for continuing education and professional development and contributes to the professional growth of others.

Rationale

The scientific, cultural, social, and political changes characterizing our contemporary society require the nurse to be committed to the ongoing pursuit of knowledge that will enhance professional growth.

Standard IX. Interdisciplinary Collaboration

The nurse collaborates with other health care providers in assessing, planning, implementing, and evaluating programs and other mental health activities.

Rationale

Psychiatric nursing requires planning and sharing with others to deliver maximum mental health services to the client and the community. Through the collaborative process, different abilities of health care providers are utilized to communicate, plan, solve problems, and evaluate services delivered.

Standard X. Utilization of Community Health Systems

The nurse participates with other members of the community in assessing, planning, implementing, and evaluating mental health services and community systems that include the promotion of the broad continuum of primary, secondary, and tertiary prevention of mental illness.

Rationale

The high incidence of mental illness in our contemporary society requires increased effort to devise more effective treatment and prevention programs. Nurses must participate in programs that strengthen the existing health potential of all members of society. Such concepts as primary prevention and continuity of care are essential in planning to meet the mental health needs of the community. The nurse uses organizational, advisory, advocacy, and consultative skills to facilitate the development and implementation of mental health services.

Standard XI. Research

The nurse contributes to nursing and the mental health field through innovations in theory and practice and participation in research.

Rationale

Each professional has responsibility for the continuing development and refinement of knowledge in the mental health field through research and experimentation with new and creative approaches to practice.

Source: *Standards of Psychiatric and Mental Health Nursing Practice.* Kansas City: American Nurses Association, 1982. Used with permission.

Appendix B: NANDA Taxonomy I Revised

The North American Nursing Diagnosis Association's Taxonomy I Revised, organized around nine human response patterns, is the currently accepted classification system for nursing diagnoses. The nine human response patterns are exchanging, communicating, relating, valuing, choosing, moving, perceiving, knowing, and feeling.

The complete taxonomic structure is listed below. Note that a series of numbers precedes each diagnosis. Each new diagnosis approved by NANDA is assigned a classification number. This number is used to determine the placement of the new diagnosis within the taxonomy. The number of digits assigned is related to the level of abstraction of the nursing diagnosis (more specific diagnoses are assigned longer numbers). The numbering system is intended to facilitate computerization of the taxonomy.

Pattern 1. Exchanging *(Mutual giving and receiving)*

1.1.2.1	Altered nutrition: More than body requirements
1.1.2.2	Altered nutrition: Less than body requirements
1.1.2.3	Altered nutrition: Potential for more than body requirements
1.2.1.1	High risk for infection
1.2.2.1	High risk for altered body temperature
1.2.2.2	Hypothermia
1.2.2.3	Hyperthermia
1.2.2.4	Ineffective thermoregulation
1.2.3.1	Dysreflexia
1.3.1.1	Constipation
1.3.1.1.1	Perceived constipation
1.3.1.1.2	Colonic constipation
1.3.1.2	Diarrhea
1.3.1.3	Bowel incontinence
1.3.2	Altered urinary elimination
1.3.2.1.1	Stress incontinence
1.3.2.1.2	Reflex incontinence
1.3.2.1.3	Urge incontinence
1.3.2.1.4	Functional incontinence
1.3.2.1.5	Total incontinence
1.3.2.2	Urinary retention
1.4.1.1	Altered (specify type) tissue perfusion (renal, cerebral, cardiopulmonary, gastrointestinal, peripheral)

1.4.1.2.1	Fluid volume excess
1.4.1.2.2.1	Fluid volume deficit
1.4.1.2.2.2	High risk for fluid volume deficit
1.4.2.1	Decreased cardiac output
1.5.1.1	Impaired gas exchange
1.5.1.2	Ineffective airway clearance
1.5.1.3	Ineffective breathing pattern
1.5.1.3.1	Inability to sustain spontaneous ventilation
1.5.1.3.2	Dysfunctional ventilatory weaning response
1.6.1	High risk for injury
1.6.1.1	High risk for suffocation
1.6.1.2	High risk for poisoning
1.6.1.3	High risk for trauma
1.6.1.4	High risk for aspiration
1.6.1.5	High risk for disuse syndrome
1.6.2	Altered protection
1.6.2.1	Impaired tissue integrity
1.6.2.1.1	Altered oral mucous membrane
1.6.2.1.2.1	Impaired skin integrity
1.6.2.1.2.2	High risk for impaired skin integrity

Pattern 2. Communicating *(Sending messages)*

2.1.1.1	Impaired verbal communication

Pattern 3. Relating *(Establishing bonds)*

3.1.1	Impaired social interaction
3.1.2	Social isolation
3.2.1	Altered role performance
3.2.1.1.1	Altered parenting
3.2.1.1.2	High risk for altered parenting
3.2.1.2.1	Sexual dysfunction
3.2.2	Altered family processes
3.2.2.1	Caregiver role strain
3.2.2.2	High risk for caregiver role strain
3.2.3.1	Parental role conflict
3.3	Altered sexuality patterns

Pattern 4. Valuing *(Assigning relative worth)*

4.1.1	Spiritual distress (distress of the human spirit)

Pattern 5. Choosing *(Selecting alternatives)*

5.1.1.1	Ineffective individual coping
5.1.1.1.1	Impaired adjustment
5.1.1.1.2	Defensive coping
5.1.1.1.3	Ineffective denial
5.1.2.1.1	Ineffective family coping: Disabling
5.1.2.1.2	Ineffective family coping: Compromised
5.1.2.2	Family coping: Potential for growth
5.2.1	Ineffective management of therapeutic regimen (individual)
5.2.1.1	Noncompliance (specify)
5.3.1.1	Decisional conflict (specify)
5.4	Health-seeking behaviors (specify)

Pattern 6. Moving *(Involving Activity)*

6.1.1.1	Impaired physical mobility
6.1.1.1.1	High risk for peripheral neurovascular dysfunction
6.1.1.2	Activity intolerance
6.1.1.2.1	Fatigue
6.1.1.3	High risk for activity intolerance
6.2.1	Sleep pattern disturbance
6.3.1.1	Diversional activity deficit
6.4.1.1	Impaired home maintenance management
6.4.2	Altered health maintenance
6.5.1	Feeding self-care deficit
6.5.1.1	Impaired swallowing
6.5.1.2	Ineffective breast-feeding
6.5.1.2.1	Interrupted breast-feeding
6.5.1.3	Effective breast-feeding
6.5.1.4	Ineffective infant feeding pattern
6.5.2	Bathing/hygiene self-care deficit
6.5.3	Dressing/grooming self-care deficit
6.5.4	Toileting self-care deficit
6.6	Altered growth and development
6.7	Relocation stress syndrome

Pattern 7. Perceiving *(Receiving information)*

7.1.1	Body image disturbance
7.1.2	Self-esteem disturbance
7.1.2.1	Chronic low self-esteem
7.1.2.2	Situational low self-esteem

7.1.3	Personal identity disturbance
7.2	Sensory/perceptual alterations (specify—visual, auditory, kinesthetic, gustatory, tactile, olfactory)
7.2.1.1	Unilateral neglect
7.3.1	Hopelessness
7.3.2	Powerlessness

Pattern 8. Knowing *(Associating meaning with information)*

8.1.1	Knowledge deficit (specify)
8.3	Altered thought processes

Pattern 9. Feeling *(Being subjectively aware of information)*

9.1.1	Pain
9.1.1.1	Chronic pain
9.2.1.1	Dysfunctional grieving
9.2.1.2	Anticipatory grieving
9.2.2	High risk for violence: Self-directed or directed at others
9.2.2.1	High risk for self-mutilation
9.2.3	Posttrauma response
9.2.3.1	Rape-trauma syndrome
9.2.3.1.1	Rape-trauma syndrome: Compound reaction
9.2.3.1.2	Rape-trauma syndrome: Silent reaction
9.3.1	Anxiety
9.3.2	Fear

Appendix C: Normal values for common laboratory tests

Electrolyte levels

Sodium: 135 to 145 mEq/liter

Potassium: 3.5 to 5 mEq/liter

Calcium: 9 to 10.5 mg/dl

Arterial blood gas analysis

PaO_2: 75 to 100 mm Hg

$PaCO_2$: 35 to 45 mm Hg

pH: 7.35 to 7.42

O_2 saturation: 94% to 100%

HCO_3^-: 22 to 26 mEq/liter

Complete blood count

Red blood cell count: 4.2 to 6 million/mm^3

Hemoglobin level: 12 to 18 g/dl

White blood cell count: 5,000 to 10,000/mm^3

Platelet count: 150,000 to 400,000/mm^3

Erythrocyte sedimentation rate: 1 to 20 mm/hour

Other blood tests

Fasting plasma glucose test: 80 to 120 mg/dl

Serum cholesterol level: 150 to 250 mg/dl

Prothrombin time: 11 to 12.5 seconds

Clotting time: 6 to 17 minutes

Partial thromboplastin time: 30 to 40 seconds

Renal function tests

Blood urea nitrogen: 8 to 20 mg/dl

Creatinine level: 0.8 to 1.5 mg/dl

Liver function tests

Total protein: 6 to 8 g/dl

Albumin-globulin ratio
  Albumin: 3.8 to 5 g/dl
  Globulin: 2.3 to 3.5 g/dl
  A-G ratio: 1.1 to 2.1

Serum glutamic-pyruvic transaminase: 5 to 35 units/ml

Serum glutamic-oxaloacetic transaminase: 5 to 40 units/ml

Lactic dehydrogenase: 200 to 450 units/ml

Alkaline phosphatase: 1.5 to 4 Bodansky units/dl or 4 to 13.5 King-Armstrong units/dl

Serum bilirubin: less than 1 mg/dl

Selected references

Applebaum, P., et al. *Informed Consent: Legal Theory and Clinical Practice.* New York: Oxford University Press, 1987.

Barnum, B.S. *Nursing Theory: Analysis, Application, Evaluation,* 3rd ed. Glennview, Ill.: Scott, Foresman & Co., 1990.

Benner, M.P. *Mental Health and Psychiatric Nursing,* 2nd ed. Springhouse, Pa.: Springhouse Corp., 1993.

Boyd, C.O. "Qualitative Approaches to Nursing Research," in *Nursing Research: Principles and Methods.* Philadelphia: J.B. Lippincott, 1990.

Burges, A. *Psychiatric Nursing in the Hospital and Community,* 5th ed. Norwalk, Conn.: Appleton & Lange, 1991.

Calfee, B.E. "Confidentiality and Disclosure of Medical Information," *Nursing Management* 20(12): 20-23, December 1989.

Carmines, E.G., and Zeller, R.A. *Reliability and Validity Assessment.* Newbury Park, Calif.: Sage University Press, 1989.

Cohen, S., and Callahan, J. *The Diagnosis and Treatment of Drug and Alcohol Abuse.* New York: Haworth Press, 1986.

Corey, E., et al. "Psychodynamic Nursing," in *Nursing Theorists and Their Works.* Edited by Marriner, A. St. Louis: C.V. Mosby, 1986.

Craig, S., et al. "Seclusion and Restraint: Decreasing the Discomfort," *Journal of Psychosocial Nursing* 27(7): 16-19, July 1989.

Diagnostic and Statistical Manual of Mental Disorders, 3rd ed., rev. New York: American Psychiatric Association, 1987.

Doenges, M., and Moorhous, M. *Nursing Diagnoses with Interventions,* 3rd ed. Philadelphia: F.A. Davis, 1991.

Dubrul, T. "Separation-Individuation Roller Coaster in the Therapy of a Borderline Patient," *Perspectives in Psychiatric Care* 25(3-4): 10-14, March-April, 1989.

Erickson, E. *Childhood and Society.* New York: W.W. Norton & Co., 1950.

Fawcett, J. *Conceptual Models of Nursing,* 2nd ed. Philadelphia: F.A. Davis, 1989.

Faye, G., and Kavanaugh, C. *Psychiatric Mental Health Nursing.* Philadelphia: J.B. Lippincott, 1990.

Fiesta, J. *The Law and Liability: A Guide for Nurses,* 2nd ed. New York: John Wiley & Sons, 1988.

Forchuk, C., and Brown, B. "Establishing a Nurse-Client Relationship," *Journal of Psychosocial Nursing* 27(2): 30-34, February 1989.

Forchuk, C., et al. "Incorporating Peplau's Theory and Case Management," *Journal of Psychosocial Nursing* 27(2): 35-38, February 1989.

Gary, F., and Kavanagh, C. *Psychiatric Mental Health Nursing.* St. Louis: J.B. Lippincott, 1991.

Ginsburg, H., and Opper, S. *Piaget's Theory of Intellectual Development.* Englewood Cliffs, N.J.: Prentice-Hall, 1969.

Haber, J., et al. *Comprehensive Psychiatric Nursing,* 3rd ed. New York: McGraw-Hill Book Co., 1987.

Keltner, N., et al. *Psychiatric Nursing: A Psychotherapeutic Management Approach.* St. Louis: Mosby Year-Book, 1991.

Knapp, S., and VandeCreek, L. *Privileged Communication in the Mental Health Professions.* New York: Von Nostrand Reinhold Co., 1987.

LoBiondo-Wood, G., and Haber, J. *Nursing Research: Methods, Critical Appraisal, and Utilization,* 2nd ed. St. Louis: C.V. Mosby Co., 1990.

McFarland, G., and Thomas, M. *Psychiatric Mental Health Nursing: Application of the Nursing Process.* St. Louis: J.B. Lippincott, 1991.

Munro, B.H., et al. *Statistical Methods for Health Care Research.* Philadelphia: J.B. Lippincott, 1986.

Nehls, N. "Borderline Personality Disorder and Group Therapy," *Archives of Psychiatric Nursing* 5(3): 137-146, March 1991.

Norris, J., et al. *Mental Health-Psychiatric Nursing: A Continuum of Care.* New York: John Wiley & Sons, 1987.

Northrop, C.E., and Kelly, M.E. *Legal Issues in Nursing.* St. Louis: C.V. Mosby Co., 1987.

Piaget, J. "Stages of the Intellectual Development of the Child," *Bulletin of the Menninger Clinic* 26(4103): 120-132, 1962.

Piccinino, S. "The Nursing Care Challenge: Borderline Patients," *Journal of Psychosocial Nursing* 28(4): 22-27, April 1990.

Polit, D.F., and Hungler, B.P. *Nursing Research: Principles and Methods,* 4th ed. Philadelphia: J.B. Lippincott, 1991.

Runyon, N., et al. "The Borderline Patient on the Med-Surg Unit, *American Journal of Nursing* 88(12): 1644-1649, December 1988.

Strauss, A., and Corbin, J. *Basics of Qualitative Research: Grounded Theory Procedures and Techniques.* Newbury Park, Calif.: Sage University Press, 1990.

Stuart. G., and Surdeen, S. *Principles and Practice of Psychiatric Nursing,* 4th ed. St. Louis: C.V. Mosby Co., 1991.

Townsend, M.C. *Nursing Diagnosis in Psychiatric Nursing.* Philadelphia: F.A. Davis, 1989.

Varcarolis, E. *Foundations of Mental Health Nursing.* Philadelphia: W.B. Saunders Co, 1990.

Webster, C. "Managing the Borderline Personality," *Nursing Management* 20(2): 49-51, February 1989.

Webster, J. "Rethinking Inpatient Treatment of Borderline Clients," *Perspectives in Psychiatric Care* 27(2): 17-20, February 1991.

Index

t refers to a table.

t refers to a table.

t refers to a table.